AROMATHERAPY AND MASSAGE FOR PEOPLE WITH LEARNING DIFFICULTIES

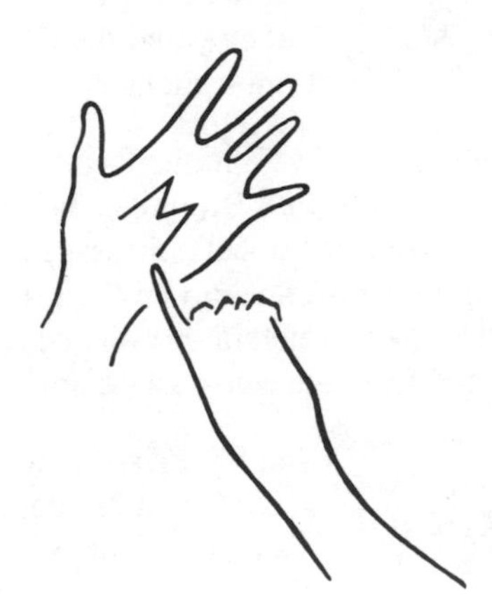

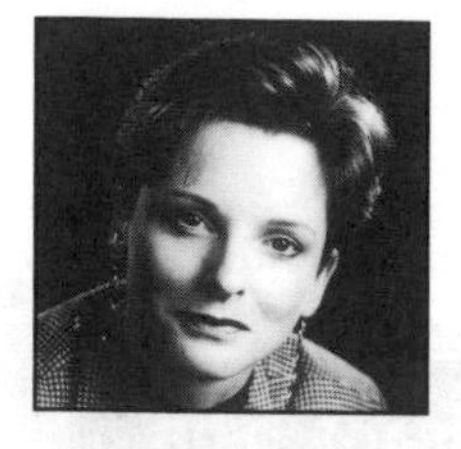

Helen Sanderson trained as an occupational therapist and has worked with people who have learning difficulties in day centres, a hospital, and in the community. She became interested in aromatherapy through her work, qualified as an aromatherapist and introduced its use with people who have learning difficulties.

Living in Manchester, Helen now works as a development officer for Social Services. She has a private aromatherapy practice, has written many articles, and contributed to books and training packages in addition to teaching aromatherapy courses.

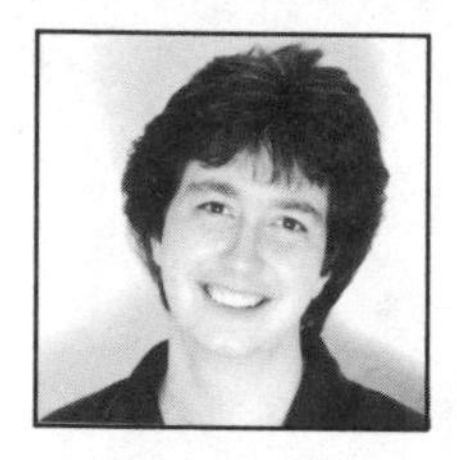

Jane Harrison has worked for many years with people with learning difficulties. Her particular interest in supporting people with multiple disabilities and challenging behaviour led her to Germany where she studied Prekop's Holding Therapy and the educational healing work of Rudolf Steiner.

After completing an M.A. in the Psychology of Mental Handicap, Jane spent six years with Birmingham Social Services. During this time she trained in therapeutic massage at the College of Holistic Medicine in London. She now lives in Birmingham and offers massage therapy at a natural health centre and at Sense-In-The-Midlands and facilitates workshops around the country and abroad.

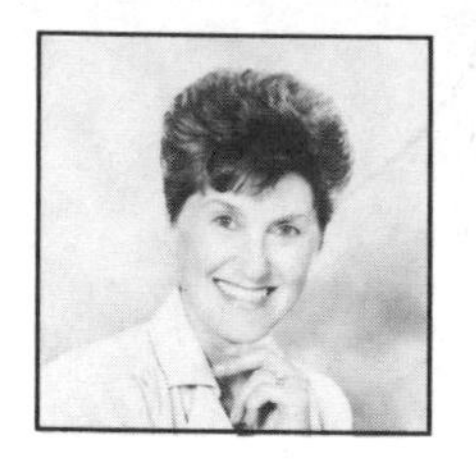

Shirley Price is an internationally recognised authority on aromatherapy. This is her third book on the subject, the first two successes being "Practical Aromatherapy" and "Aromatherapy for Common Ailments"; her fourth book "The Shirley Price Aromatherapy Workbook" covers aromatherapy in greater depth.

Much of Shirley's time is spent lecturing throughout the UK and abroad on behalf of aromatherapy, to encourage its use in hospitals and to bring it within reach of the lay person in a safe and usable fashion. At home she oversees the development of her flourishing aromatherapy organisation.

WA 1201059 6

AROMATHERAPY AND MASSAGE FOR PEOPLE WITH LEARNING DIFFICULTIES

GLYNTAFF

UNIVERSITY OF GLAMORGAN
LEARNING RESOURCES CENTRE

Pontypridd, Mid Glamorgan, CF37 1DL
Telephone: Pontypridd (01443) 482626

Books are to be returned on or before the last date below

ONE WEEK LOAN

13 JULY '01

Printed and bound
in Great Britain by
The Abbott Press Limited
Lutterworth
Leicestershire

First published
in the United Kingdom by
Hands On Publishing
62 Sir Johns Road
Selly Park
Birmingham
B29 7ER
© 1991

Helen Sanderson, Jane Harrison and Shirley Price
Re-printed 1993
Re-printed 1994
Re-printed 1995
Re-printed 1996
Re-printed 1997
Re-printed 1998
Re-printed 1999

All rights reserved
No part of this publication may be reproduced,
stored in a retrieval system or transmitted,
in any form or by any means, without the prior
permission in writing of the publisher, nor be
otherwise circulated in any form of binding or cover
other than that in which it is published and without
a similar condition, including this condition,
being imposed upon the purchaser.

The right of
Helen Sanderson, Jane Harrison and Shirley Price
to be identified as the authors of this work
has been asserted in accordance with Sections 77 and 78
of the Copyright, Designs and Patents Act 1988,
United Kingdom.

The techniques, ideas and suggestions in this book
are not intended as a substitute for proper medical advice.
Any application of the techniques, ideas and suggestions
in this book is at the readers' sole discretion and risk.

ISBN 0-9518172-0-5

12010596

Contents

Acknowledgements

Without the people with learning difficulties and their advocates who have experienced and supported our work, these ideas would not have been developed and this book could not have been written.

Our sincere thanks to all who have taught us so much.

We are also indebted to a number of people who have been invaluable for their support, enthusiasm, comments, contributions of their experiences, typing and proof-reading.

Thank you to:

John Aston, Pat Berry, Margaret Bisset, Sue Carmichael, Maureen Farrell, Margaret Firth, Sarah Fitzgerald, Nicola Hyde-Gitsham, Andrew Gitsham, Sylvia Gitsham, Marci Green, Maureen Hanse, Jo Helas, Jane Holden, Michael McGarry, Rose Martin, Lynn McCulloch, Sue Menzies, John Oliver, Elaine Reader, Hazel Reyndesh, Judy Ruddle, Carolyn Sanderson, Jane Turnbull, Mark Warren, and to Sylvia Baker and Justine Finney at S.P.A. Ltd.

We would like to thank Ken Eyerman and his publishers, Sidgwick and Jackson, for allowing us to quote from his book ''Massage'' at the beginning of Chapter 18.

A special thank you also to:

All those who have participated in the course, 'Aromatherapy and Massage for People who have Learning Difficulties' for sharing our enthusiasm.

For uniformity we have used 'she' or 'her' throughout the text instead of he/she, his/her.

Introduction

The principle of 'ordinary lives for ordinary people', which is encompassed by the Five Accomplishments (O'Brien, J. 1986), and the holistic, individual-based approach of aromatherapy and massage, provide the firm values base from which we have approached our work and written this book.

The best place for us all to thrive, learn and develop is in an environment where each one of us is respected as a person with individual physical, emotional, intellectual and spiritual traits and needs. Aromatherapy and massage can touch and connect each of those parts and can also help to create a supportive, positive and stimulating environment in which the particular needs of each individual may be met.

The following chapters discuss how aromatherapy and massage can be used to relax, invigorate and improve the health of people who have learning difficulties. However, massage does not only have to be a passive activity luxuriously received by those who can afford it. In this book we have developed two other forms of massage which can be used by anyone and which are appropriate to the individual needs of people who have severe and profound learning difficulties.

Interactive Massage

This approach emphasises the way in which massage can help to develop communication, trust and interaction in a non-verbal and non- threatening way, enabling individuals to become more aware of other people as well as themselves. In Interactive Massage the emphasis is on encouraging the person to respond and participate, guided by the stages of the Interactive Sequence (McInnes and Treffry, 1982).

Multisensory Massage

Multisensory Massage can be either passive or interactive in nature, with the emphasis being on increasing the person's awareness of the environment through tactile and olfactory stimulation using different textures and smells within massage.

As an aromatherapist and a massage therapist who work with people both with and without learning difficulties, we find that the beneficial effects of aromatherapy and massage are the same for everyone.

It therefore follows that there are no special 'remedies' specific to people who have learning difficulties, and the basic principles described here are applicable to anybody.

However, we would like to offer our experience and ideas which are based on the ways in which we have used aromatherapy and massage successfully in day centres, schools, hospitals and community settings.

In most chapters we have included sections entitled 'Theory into Practice'. These are real examples of how aromatherapy and massage have been used by ourselves and others with people who have learning difficulties.

Experienced aromatherapists and massage therapists can offer a depth of knowledge and experience, but *anybody* can introduce aromatherapy and massage into the lives of the people they support. We hope that through this book more people will be encouraged to try out and sample the benefits of these two ancient therapies.

1

The Sense of Touch

The information which we receive from our senses of sight, hearing, touch, taste and smell is vital to enable us to understand our environment. Carol Ouvry (1987) states that "sensory perception provides the information upon which children base their understanding of the surroundings which guide their responses to the environment."

It is well known that people who suffer the loss of one of their senses experience compensation through the development of the other remaining senses. Due to sensory impairment or lack of opportunity, people who have more severe and profound learning difficulties are often unable to gather, interpret and respond to sensory information. Aromatherapy and massage can enable people to become more aware and appreciative of their senses of touch and smell.

■ The Importance of Touch

"Touch is a basic behavioural need, in much the same way as breathing is a basic physical need. When the need for touch remains unsatisfied abnormal behaviour will result" (Montague, A. 1986).

The importance of touch for both physical and mental health has been the subject of much interest and research. The absence of touch has been shown to have profound effects on health. Gentle handling of rats makes the difference between life and death following the removal of significant endocrine glands. In addition to these effects on health, the absence of touch can have profound effects on behaviour. Handling or 'gentling' of rats produced gentle, unexcitable animals, whereas lack of 'gentling' resulted in frightened, nervous and agitated rats (Montague, A. 1986). Similar results were recorded in Harlow's famous monkey experiments where infant monkeys raised in a cage with a bare wire mesh floor survived with difficulty, whilst infant monkeys who were given a wire mesh cone covered in towelling representing a mother substitute, thrived (Harlow, H.F. 1965).

It is known that premature babies thrive, and children in hospital recover more quickly, if touched and cuddled. Dr Rene Spitz of the New York Foundling Hospital found that although babies in the hospital were kept well fed and in clean conditions, they had a high death rate. Holidaying in Mexico, Dr Spitz observed babies in a local orphanage, not so clean and well-fed, but nevertheless happier and healthier than those in the Foundling Hospital. The difference lay in the fact that the village women came into the orphanage every day and played with the children. They fondled, stroked and talked to the babies, while in New York, the children were left in their cots (Spitz, R. 1946).

Dr James Prescot, an American neuropsychologist states that the absence or withdrawal of physical affection in early life, and even as an adult, may be responsible for many types of disturbed behaviour such as depression, violence, aggression and hyperactivity (Prescot, J. 1963). In one hospital, disturbed teenagers go through an intensive course of physical treatment, learning to appreciate the significance of touching and being touched. Since this kind of therapy has been introduced, violence at the hospital has noticeably abated (Hooper, A. 1988).

Could it be that a lack of touch contributes to the challenging behaviours exhibited by some people who have learning difficulties? Self-stimulatory behaviours may be a result of insufficient tactile stimulation (McCray, G. 1978). Rocking behaviour, for example, represents a kind of self comfort, which is also seen in people who are grieving and mourning. Shevrin and Toussieng (1965) suggest that rocking is used as a form of tactile behaviour where touching is absent. Provence and Lipton (1962) compared the behaviour of institutionalised infants and infants who live with families. They found that the institutionalised infants reacted strangely to being held and displayed rocking behaviour.

Hogg, Sebba, and Lambe (1990) suggest that as the normal pleasures of touching and being touched for its own sake are not readily available to an individual with severe and profound learning difficulties, she may consequently seek more accessible tactile stimuli. This may include head banging and other forms of self-mutilation, body rocking, frequent masturbation or physical aggression. "The individual may learn to associate physical contact with another person with unpleasant, painful or perfunctory experiences and become tactile defensive, rejecting contact out of hand.''

How should this convincing evidence of the effects of lack of touch affect our interactions with people who have learning difficulties?

■ Touch as Communication

Touch is a universal language, a way of connecting, exchanging information and communicating. We give and receive many messages through touch;

I need comforting
I am here
I'm in pain
Come here, I'll rub it better
I need reassurance
You're doing really well
I feel comfortable with you

Gently holding a hand, a kind touch on the arm, a pat on the back or holding someone who is crying can often convey silently but more clearly and easily than words how people really feel.

Touch is central to our work with people who have severe learning difficulties, yet the issues it raises are rarely addressed and clarified. Our professional or supportive role involves much functional touching, taking people to the toilet, washing them, dressing them, possibly moving them in and out of wheelchairs. Yet many struggle with issues around the ''appropriateness'' of hugging an adult or having her sit on a lap. Whilst recognising the importance of touch, how can we ensure that we touch people with learning difficulties in an age- appropriate and respectful manner? This issue can be addressed by considering the quality of the touch which people receive in everyday interactions, and the use of massage.

The Quality of Touch

For people who have severe or profound learning difficulties, and particularly those who have dual sensory impairment, touch may be the clearest way that people have of understanding the world, communicating their needs and receiving information from the people around them.

Anita Royall writes of the importance of having a ''multisensory approach (which) aims to use all the child's senses to break through the barrier of a child's handicap and communicate with the child.''

The quality of touch which a person receives is therefore very important. Touch can be affirming and supportive. It can also be rough and manipulative. A rough movement or irritable push even if accompanied by words of encouragement, will show how you are really feeling and will make the person feel spurned rather than supported. In a therapeutic environment where people with learning difficulties are learning new skills, taking risks and developing independence, their perception of themselves as able, valued and developing people is crucial. That self worth will only grow if the support worker is able to transmit genuine feelings of encouragement, respect and even excitement about the development of that person. As Flo Longhorn (1988) says: ''The quality of the touch can dictate the success or failure of the session and of the relationship.''

Our touch therefore, should be facilitative not forceful, respectful not abusive and receptive to the person not manipulative. A person who trusts, feels safe and reassured will learn more readily than one who is frightened, detached and unresponsive. By taking time to consider the quality of touch we give, we can affect not only the quality of our relationships with the people we support but also the quality of their lives.

Touch and Massage

Massage is an appropriate, valued way of incorporating touch into a person's life at home or in a learning environment. It is easy to learn and wonderful to do.

Some people may be concerned about the sexual implications of massage. Our experience is that if the touch communicated through massage is not intended to be sexual, then it will usually be perceived as non-sexual. You can reduce the likelihood of misunderstanding by avoiding particularly sensitive areas, being clear about the intention of the massage and choosing carefully who massages whom.

Massage has a long and health-promoting history. It is one of the oldest and simplest of medical treatments. In some cultures, particularly in the East, it is accepted as natural that people of all ages benefit from regular massage. Indeed, in China, massage is often the first treatment for most childhood illnesses.

Here in the West we have tended to underestimate the power of touch, and the value of massage has only recently become more recognised. All too often we tend to be afraid to touch one another. Yet as we have shown, research continues to demonstrate how extraordinarily effective touch can be, and touch is the core of massage.

Massage is an extension of touch, an extension of the natural urge to rub something better. Professional massage treatment now comes in a variety of forms - Therapeutic massage, Aromatherapy, Reflexology, Shiatsu, Rolfing, Biodynamic massage, Touch for Health and many more. However, massage does not have to be complicated to be effective. Stroking a baby's brow will send her to sleep; massaging a hand can soothe a frightened child or distressed patient; partners can share massage to develop their relationship and relax each other. At a more advanced therapeutic level many common ailments such as headaches, back pain or arthritis can be helped by massage.

Massage is well known for its relaxing effects or treatment of sports injuries but regular massage will go further than this and improve overall health. By relaxing the muscles and stimulating the circulation of blood and lymph, toxins and waste that limit the healthy functioning of the body are expelled and the person's digestion, breathing and posture will improve. As the body starts to change and heal, the feelings of irritability, fear, anxiety or depression that so often accompany the physical symptoms are also dispelled, restoring a sense of wholeness and revitalisation.

Massage has a wide range of applications and benefits which are available to people who have learning difficulties. Whether in everyday contact or channelled into a therapy such as massage, touch is an important part of our lives. The issues it raises are challenging and also central to the way we relate to others. By rising to the challenge of providing affirming and appropriate touch, we can significantly improve the effectiveness of the time we spend supporting people with learning difficulties, thus making it more enjoyable and meaningful.

2

The Sense of Smell

The sense of smell is perhaps the most under-used sense and yet it is 10,000 times more sensitive than that of taste. In the animal kingdom it plays a vital role in survival. Animals rely on their sense of smell to identify territory, locate food and recognise each other. The sense of smell is less developed in humans and has a slight protective function. It can alert people to rotten food, poisonous fumes or fire and continues to function during sleep when most of our other senses are dulled.

Although the sense of smell is not as developed in us as in many species of animals, the human nose can still identify up to 400,000 different odours. This accuracy is dulled by illness, particularly when suffering from infections of the respiratory tract such as colds or 'flu.

Robert Tisserand (1988) describes how astronauts suffered from olfactory deprivation during the initial long term space flights as they had nothing except lemon scented hand wipes to smell. These were soon saved for sniffing sessions and became valued items. During later flights astronauts carried bottled reproductions of familiar smells and scented items to help prevent homesickness.

The sense of smell is often not considered to be clinically important; yet an individual with profound learning difficulties, if not encouraged to use this sense, lacks another avenue from which to gain information and awareness of the environment.

■ How the Sense of Smell Develops

From birth, whilst their eyesight is still poor, babies rely on their sense of smell to seek their mothers milk. It used to be thought that very young children were unable to distinguish between smells, finding all odours acceptable. However, recent studies conducted by a psychologist in Philadelphia suggest otherwise. A number of nine month old babies were given scented rattles to play with and their reactions were recorded on video. It was found that the babies responded negatively to the rattle fragranced with smelly feet and favourably to a wintergreen fragrance (The International Journal of Aromatherapy, Vol.2, No.2, 1990).

Danielle Ryman (1984) suggests that children largely learn to discriminate between 'good' and 'bad' smells from the reactions of their parents and peers. She describes how young children have been shown to be highly attracted to the smell of strawberries and vanilla. From the age of 10, children develop a liking for musk and orange as well as strawberries. As the sense of smell matures and becomes more sophisticated, people begin to discriminate between different pleasant fragrances and identify their favourites. Where two fragrances are generally considered to be pleasantly acceptable, for example lavender and geranium, an individual may like one and dislike the other.

Recent research on odour preferences suggests that extroverts tend to prefer lighter fragrances and introverts the heavier, oriental scents (Lake, M. 1990).

Some researchers and aromatherapists suggest that more attention should be given to developing a greater awareness of the sense of smell, particularly during school years. In order to move some way towards this, a day has been set aside specifically to encourage people to become more aware of their sense of smell. 'World Smell Day' is on the 16th of June every year.

Flo Longhorn, in her book 'A Sensory Curriculum for Very Special People' (1988), describes how a 'Smell Curriculum' and 'Smell Bank' could be developed at school. She suggests that for children with profound learning difficulties smelling is not a passive or isolated process: "It is of little use to place a child near a vase of flowers and expect him to smell them. You must position the child comfortably, bring the flowers up to his nose, tell him what he is smelling and let him touch them."

A large proportion of taste is actually smell. Working with children to develop their awareness of the sense of smell has often resulted in improved eating skills. In the Smell Curriculum, children are encouraged to respond to pleasant and unpleasant smells. Many children who initially appear indifferent to a range of pleasant smells, learn to respond to them, develop preferences and indicate their favourites. A 'Smell Bank' is an area of the classroom which is designated as the learning area for smell, where different smells are stored in a trolley or cupboard. A range of essential oils can play a valuable role in any 'Smell Bank'. As children identify their favourites these can be used in the home to fragrance rooms and clothing, and added to the bath. Massage oils or lotions can be made with the child's favourite essential oil and used for Multisensory Massage (see Chapter 11).

Once an individual who has profound learning difficulties has learned to discriminate between different smells, it is then possible for her to choose her own fragrance or perfume.

Theory into Practice

Jean, who is 24 and is described as having a profound learning difficulty and a visual handicap, appeared to indicate a preference for a particular fragrance. Jean repeatedly turned her head towards one fragrance whilst turning her head away from others which were presented to her. This was then used to scent her clothes by impregnating a handkerchief with the oil and putting it in her drawer. The same oil was used in a burner in her bedroom of the hostel in which she lived.

It was hoped that by using a fragrance which Jean liked in her room, her clothes and her bath, she would gradually learn to identify things which were her own. The fragrance was an expression of her choice and could contribute to her sense of identity.

■ The Process of Smelling

On the inside of the nose lies a thin mucus membrane into which filaments, known as 'olfactory hairs' project. These filaments or hairs 'catch' odour molecules and affect the nerve cells which transmit impulses to the limbic system of the brain, via the olfactory nerves. Research done by the Olfaction Research Group at Warwick University has revealed that there is little doubt that the olfactory system directly targets the limbic area of the brain which is concerned with both motor functions and emotional expression (Van Toller, S. Dodd, G. 1988).

This suggests that essential oils can affect emotions and motor functions through their fragrance.

The nose can only respond to 3-4 smells one after another, after which a process known as 'tiring' occurs, when the nose is no longer as sensitive to the odour. This is important to consider when encouraging a person to choose a smell. It is best to offer a maximum of 3 different fragrances at any one time to prevent tiring occurring.

The process of smelling can be affected by certain chemicals contained in some air fresheners called 'Malodour Counteractants'. These act on the olfactory nerves to stimulate the sense of smell so that it reacts more strongly to the product's fragrance than that of the offensive smell. One G.P. has identified 51 cases where this chemical has produced reactions ranging from sleeplessness to nausea (The International Journal of Aromatherapy, Vol. 2, No. 2, 1990).

The Sense of Smell and Memory

The limbic system is often described as the 'emotional centre of the brain'. It is therefore not surprising that research has shown that smell memories can last longer than visual memories. For people who have severe learning difficulties and a visual impairment, smells can be used to enable people to identify their location. By using the same smell or scent in a particular area, it may enable people to identify where they are and so increase the likelihood of them anticipating the events which usually happen there. It is obviously important to keep these smells as naturally occurring as possible. For example, a bathroom may often smell of pine because of the cleaning agents used there. It is possible to make that scent slightly stronger and more recognisable by putting essential oil of pine on the radiator in a saucer of water.

Jane Sanderson Turnbull (1990) describes how in the school where she teaches, each member of staff wears a fabric bracelet impregnated with a particular perfume oil. The children who have profound learning difficulties are encouraged to identify staff by their sense of smell.

■ The Sense of Smell and Emotion

Smelling a fragrance or odour will not just recreate visual images of the past but also the emotions felt at that time. For some people, smelling their grandfather's tobacco or their mother's perfume will be comforting and soothing. Research at Warwick University has shown that if a new and unfamiliar smell is experienced when a person is feeling a particular emotion then, when that new smell is encountered again, the same emotion will also be felt.

This principle can be used to help people to relax in different environments. If essential oil of lavender is used regularly in massage and relaxation sessions, during which the person feels calm and relaxed, then burning the same oil in situations where the person feels upset could have calming and relaxing effects because of the unconscious emotions stimulated by that particular smell. Work in Italy with people who have mental health problems has demonstrated that more improvement is made when pleasant odours are used rather than unpleasant ones (Rovesti, P. 1971). Therefore, wherever possible, a person should be encouraged to select her favourite essential oil from the range of relaxing oils.

The results of the experiment at Warwick University also indicate that, although the nose gets used to or 'tires' of different aromas after a while, this does not decrease the effectiveness of essential oils. The fragrance used in the experiment was diluted to such an extent that it was imperceptible to the subjects, yet they still responded to it (Van Toller, S. Dodd, G. 1988).

Fragrance companies have used this principle to their advantage and tests have shown that when two racks of identical tights were put into a store, one rack impregnated with an unnoticeable trace of perfume, more tights were sold from the perfumed rack than the other. Similarly the stress levels of test subjects were measurably raised when a weak concentration of 'the smell of hospitals' (which was too dilute to be consciously perceived) was sprayed into their comfortable environment.

Aromas, emotions, memory and physical sensations are therefore linked. Smelling newly baked bread makes us feel hungry, smelling decaying food can make us nauseous and fragrances attached to different people and places can recreate many different emotions. The powerful link between aromas, memory and emotion is utilised in the 'coma kit' which is used by doctors to stimulate coma patients and bring them back to consciousness. On one occasion a man was awakened from a coma when his dog, who had been fretting at his master's absence, was brought into the hospital. The familiar smell of his beloved animal provided the trigger which brought him back to consciousness.

3

Approaching Aromatherapy and Massage from a Values Framework

Over the past twenty to thirty years there have been many changes in the services which are provided to support people who have learning difficulties. From living in large institutions people with learning difficulties are now moving back into the community and, through the emergence of the self advocacy movement, are learning to speak up for themselves. As a result of this there is a move away from the label 'mentally handicapped' to the preferred term 'people with learning difficulties'.

As people who are involved in the lives of those who have learning difficulties, whether as therapists, teachers, support workers or parents, we make daily decisions aimed at improving the quality of an individual's life.

John O'Brien (1986) suggests five key areas of experience which affect the quality of a person's life. These key areas or accomplishments consist of making choices for yourself, sharing ordinary places and activities in the community, being treated with respect, developing abilities and growing in personal relationships. O'Brien suggests that when planning activities with people who have learning difficulties we should think carefully about how each of these areas can be developed to improve the quality of that person's life. The following sections discuss how each accomplishment can be promoted using aromatherapy and massage.

■ Choice

People with learning difficulties often have limited opportunities to express their needs and make their wishes known. This may range from everyday decisions such as what to eat or what to wear, to major life changing decisions such as where to live and with whom.

When using aromatherapy and massage an emphasis should be placed on encouraging the person to choose which essential oil she prefers, when and where the massage should take place, on which parts of the body she would like to be massaged and most importantly, whether she wants a massage at all. For example, when working with a person to encourage her to relax, she could choose whether to have her hands or feet massaged, and when offered three relaxing essential oils could choose her favourite aroma to be made up into a massage oil. On some occasions, a person may not want a massage and even though you may have planned it, her right to choose must be respected.

Everyone is an individual and people who have profound or multiple disabilities may need extra support to identify their individual preferences. Research has indicated that people who have profound learning difficulties commonly look, turn and reach towards things that they like. If you are not sure how a person responds to something she likes, as opposed to something she dislikes, your speech therapist may be able to work with you using an assessment such as the Affective Communication Assessment (Coupe et al, 1985), to help you identify behaviour which indicates a positive choice.

If you offer a person three different oils slowly, one after another, you may be able to discern subtle changes. Perhaps the person may sniff one particular oil intently, push one essential oil away or reach out for another one. In choosing which area to massage you may find that the person appears to relax more quickly when you massage the feet rather than the hands.

Although it may take more time, you will find that most people with more profound learning difficulties do have definite preferences. An important aspect of the area of choice is to ensure that the person has opportunities to make informed choices. This may mean that several options are tried before the person makes a decision or informed choice. Sometimes people may refuse things which they have never experienced and in some situations may need encouragement to try different activities. If the first time you ever went to the cinema you disliked the film it would, one hopes, not prevent you from going again. In the same way two or three 'tastes' of an activity may be necessary before a person can decide. With people who have profound and multiple disabilities the Interactive Sequence (see Chapter 10) illustrates how a person may at first resist new activities, but may come to tolerate and later enjoy them.

Community Presence

On a fundamental level this means bringing people back home from hospitals and hostels, and encouraging and supporting them to live in their own homes. Community presence does not refer only to where an individual lives but also to sharing public amenities including leisure facilities, public transport, schools and public buildings. This means avoiding segregated residential, educational or leisure facilities where there are only people who have learning difficulties. Such segregated facilities keep people with learning difficulties away from other people when, with appropriate support, they can use the same services and resources as everyone else.

Usually people who would like a massage go to a natural health clinic, beauty salon, sports centre or visit an aromatherapist or massage therapist at his or her own home. Sometimes massage therapists or aromatherapists visit a person in her own home or friends may simply help each other to relax through massage. As often as possible people who have learning difficulties should use the same venues in the community as everyone else.

To find an aromatherapist or massage therapist in your area contact the training schools listed at the back of the book. Some therapists advertise in local health food shops or magazines. Check that the person is qualified with a diploma and that he or she is a member of an independent professional body such as the International Society of Professional Aromatherapists. Enquire whether the premises are accessible for wheelchairs if appropriate. The beauty salons and sports centres which offer massage will be listed in local directories.

If finances, support and opportunities do not regularly allow this, consideration can be given to using massage in the home, at a day centre or in a school, during for example a health care or relaxation session or as part of a sensory stimulation programme for people with more profound learning difficulties. As far as possible, emphasis should be placed on enabling the person to choose and purchase her own oils locally, provided *genuine* oils are available.

■ Respect

People who have learning difficulties are often 'devalued', treated as if they were second class citizens. It requires concentrated effort to assist them to have a valued place in community life. This will involve using language and images which present people with learning difficulties in a positive way, and working sensitively to understand and reduce behaviours and aspects of appearance which reinforce negative stereotypes about them. Some people with severe learning difficulties have 'good' reasons for inappropriate behaviour which may be the result of frustrated attempts at communication. Reducing these behaviours can only be done if the reasons for the behaviour are fully considered and more appropriate options suggested. For some behaviours perhaps the emphasis should be on educating the public to understand their prejudices.

It is important to consider whether activities are appropriate to a person's age. Touch is important for people and massage provides an age-appropriate and respected way of touching people. In massage (as in every other area of life) it is important to be aware of the need to accord dignity and respect in all environments whether that is in a community venue, at school, at home or in a day centre.

This respect should not only be reflected in the activity in which the person is involved, but also in the surroundings, in the opportunities which the person is given, and in the way that she is spoken to. When considering the activities and opportunities with a person it is important to choose those which will present that person in the most positive and valued way. Massage and aromatherapy are valued and accepted ways of relaxing - as most stress management books and courses will verify!

■ Capability

This refers to the improvement of skills which are needed for people to be able to make choices, form relationships, develop communication skills, and use services and resources in the community. It is also concerned with the availability of opportunities to practice these skills with whatever assistance is required. We will show later in the book, how aromatherapy and massage can be used to increase mobility, improve health, and develop body awareness. For people who have more profound learning difficulties, Multisensory and Interactive Massage can be used to increase a person's awareness of herself, other people and her environment.

■ Relationships

Very often individuals who have learning difficulties have unusually small social circles consisting of other people with learning difficulties, family and staff. Developing relationships involves supporting existing ties with family or friends and maximising opportunities for people to meet other, mostly 'non-handicapped' people in the community. One of the most valuable benefits of using massage, particularly with people who have more profound learning difficulties, is that it enables the person to develop or improve a trusting relationship through Interactive Massage (see Chapter 10). This provides a good basis from which to share other activities or learn other skills.

The five accomplishments, discussed above, provide a useful framework for those concerned about improving the quality of an individual's life. Two further accomplishments have also been suggested; 'individuality' and 'continuity'. Each accomplishment is closely linked, and if one is not fully considered the success of each of the others will be affected. When planning aromatherapy and massage consider how each of these accomplishments can be developed to enhance the person's quality of life.

4

The History of Aromatherapy

Aromatherapy is the use of essential oils obtained from plants to promote health and well being. Despite becoming increasingly popular, aromatherapy is not a new art. For centuries essential oils have been used for healing, in religious ceremonies and in perfumes. Aromas for love, aromas for war and aromas for prayer were all formulated for the kings and queens of ancient dynasties.

One of the oldest known medicinal works was about healing and preventative formulae using aromatic plants. It was written by an Egyptian around 1550 BC, and demonstrates the depth of contemporary knowledge on bactericides. There are also records of the use of essential oils in hot climates for sanitation. Certain essential oils were considered to be precious at that time, and the resins from frankincense and myrrh ranked in value with gold; hence the three gifts to the infant Jesus. Today three of the most costly oils are rose, jasmine and neroli.

Many ancient civilisations developed the use of aromas for religious purposes and medicine. The Egyptians used them widely, both as cosmetics and for embalming their dead to delay decomposition. As in other fields, the Egyptian knowledge was impressive and the forecast by them that the bodies they embalmed with herbs, spices and resins would last 3000 years has been accurate. Essential oils were also used extensively in Greece and Rome. Hippocrates, the Greek physician and father of medicine wrote that "the way to health is to have an aromatic bath and scented massage every day".

The crusaders who returned to Europe after long sessions of war in the Mediterranean countries were treated there with essential oils and floral waters for the inevitable wounds and diseases which they suffered. Thus it was that knowledge of this kind of medicine was brought to Europe.

In this country, during the great plagues, Charles II's doctors suggested that all householders should fumigate their rooms with aromatic essences to protect themselves. It was well known that perfumers and glove makers (who used to scent their gloves with essential oils to mask the odour of the wearer) rarely succumbed to the diseases of the day. This fact is attributed to the antibacterial properties of essential oils. Up until the nineteenth century doctors continued to fill the top of their walking sticks with aromatics to sniff before entering a house where there was an infectious disease.

In the nineteenth century chemists began to isolate some of the therapeutic components of certain essential oils. Today, some medicinal preparations are still based on, or include, components taken from essential oils. 'Karvol', inhalant capsules available from pharmacies, contains essential oils of cinnamon and pine. The essential oil of peppermint forms the basis of many preparations for soothing troubled stomachs.

It was a French chemist called Gattefosse who is credited with first coining the word 'Aromatherapy'. Whilst experimenting in a laboratory he burned his hand severely. Plunging his hand into essential oil of lavender, he was surprised to find that the burn healed in a very short time, without infection or scarring. He later spent many years researching the properties of essential oils and published the first book on Aromatherapy.

Madame Maury, a French biochemist, used massage extensively as her main method of applying essential oils. Perhaps because of the link with massage (not used with essential oils before Madame Maury) the word 'Aromatherapy' is often misinterpreted as being 'a massage using essential oils'. It must be emphasised that this is not the original meaning of the word. Aromatherapy, as Gattefosse intended, is the use of essential oils to promote health and combat infection, and massage is one of the several ways in which the oils can be effective. In France most professionals using essential oils are doctors who prescribe them for inhalation, compresses and internal use. In this country essential oils for therapeutic application are mainly used by aromatherapists and are prescribed for internal use only by medical herbalists and doctors.

5

Introduction to Essential Oils

An essential oil is a fragrant essence which is extracted from an aromatic plant. Each essential oil has different properties. Marjoram oil, for example, is known for its relaxing and soothing properties which help to promote sleep, and it is also used to relieve aches, sprains and muscular spasms. Essential oils are not only used in aromatherapy but also in food products, toiletries, cosmetics and medicinal preparations.

In the food and confectionery industry essential oils are sometimes used to give natural flavourings, such as oil of orange in orange flavoured chocolate.

The use of essential oils is and always has been greatest in the perfumery industry. Sandalwood is used as part of the fixative in many perfumes, including 'Chanel 19' and 'Opium'.

'Nostroline', a nasal decongestant available from pharmacies, contains essential oils of eucalyptus and geranium; in fact one quarter of prescriptions dispensed by community pharmacists in the United States contain extracts from plant life. From an early age we may learn about the therapeutic properties of plants, and when stung by nettles will surely look for a dock leaf!

Essential oils have many different physical and therapeutic properties. They are many times more concentrated than the herbs from which they are extracted and are therefore very powerful, needing only a few drops to give an effect on the mind or body. Essential oils are volatile and are highly flammable. They are non-greasy, highly complex chemical structures which are soluble to different degrees in various substances.

■ Physical Properties of Essential Oils

Volatility

All essential oils are volatile, meaning that they will readily evaporate into the atmosphere. The perfume industry has categorised essential oils into top, middle or base notes depending on the volatility of the components of each oil.

Top notes are the most volatile and are generally uplifting and awakening. The aroma from a top note may last for a maximum of twenty-four hours. Top notes include bergamot and lemon.

Base notes are slower to evaporate, with the aroma lasting for about a week. On the whole base notes are calming and sedative, two examples being cedarwood and ylang ylang.

Middle notes fall in between these two. They are often used to help relieve physical disorders and include juniper and rosemary.

All essential oils, however, can have effects both on the mood and the body of a person and the terms top, middle and base are important mainly in the making of a fragrance. The volatility of essential oils makes them ideal for room freshening, inhalation and creating a particular atmosphere, as they evaporate quickly and are easily inhaled.

Flammability

If using essential oils in a burner in a school, day centre or at home it is important to be aware of their flammability and, as with other flammable liquids, appropriate safety precautions are required.

Consistency

The term 'essential oil' is something of a misnomer as 'oil' suggests an oily, greasy consistency. In reality most essential oils have a consistency which resembles water rather than oil. One or two essential oils are notably thicker and more viscous, such as sandalwood.

Chemical Structure

Essential oils are highly complex chemicals comprising terpenes, esters, ketones, phenols, alcohols, lactones, aldehydes and oxides. The many therapeutic properties attributed to the essential oil of lavender are a result of the many different chemical components which form this particular oil. It is difficult, and in most cases almost impossible, to duplicate an essential oil synthetically, as the majority of essential oils contain between ten and two hundred different chemical components, of which some have not yet been identified.

Solubility

Essential oils dissolve readily in vegetable oil and alcohol, but only up to twenty per cent of an essential oil will dissolve in water. Adding essential oils to bath water will therefore leave a thin film on the surface of the water, and it is important to agitate the water well to disperse the oil thoroughly.

Essential oils easily diffuse through the skin and into the body, which makes them effective in treating both skin conditions and other physical disorders.

Colour

Natural essential oils are usually coloured. Essential oil of bergamot is light green, benzoin resinoid - reddish-brown, oil of orange - light orange, German chamomile - blue and some oils have only a hint of colour. Completely colourless essential oils indicate refinement, where part of the oil (usually the terpene) has been removed.

Penetration

Inhalation takes essential oils directly to the receptor cells at the top of the nose which register and transmit the aroma to the brain. Aromatic particles also reach the lungs via the nasal passages. Essential oils are believed to penetrate the skin via pores and hair follicles and also to permeate between the cells of the epidermis. From here they are carried by the extracellular fluids to the blood and lymph, and hence round the body. The fact that certain substances when applied externally to the skin can affect internal organs is one of the fundamentals of aromatherapy. Rubbing raw garlic onto the soles of the feet at night can result in the odour of garlic on the breath in the morning. Essential oils are usually excreted from the body after three to six hours, or longer if the person is very overweight.

■ Therapeutic Properties of Essential Oils

It is the therapeutic properties of essential oils which have led to their use for healing and to which Gattefosse applied the term 'Aromatherapy'.

These therapeutic properties are demonstrated by the fact that they are anti-inflammatory, analgesic, bactericidal, antiviral and antiseptic. These facts will be discussed in detail in Chapter 12.

Essential oils are also synergistic, which means that their effect is enhanced if two or three oils are combined. Up to five essential oils can be mixed together, but it is not recommended that a blend of more than five be used.

In addition to having these valuable therapeutic properties, aromatherapy is well known for its relaxing effects, particularly when used in combination with massage. Many books and articles on stress recommend the use of aromatherapy and massage as ways of combating tension and promoting relaxation.

Less attention is given to the invigorating and refreshing properties of different essentials oils which can help relieve fatigue and improve concentration. Some essential oils have been found to have normalising or balancing effects, eg. geranium, lavender, clary sage.

The aroma and quality of pure essential oils from the same field may vary from harvest to harvest depending on the weather, the soil and the general climate of the area in which the plants have been grown, as does wine.

■ Extraction of Essential Oils

Depending on the plant, essential oils are found in the flowers (neroli), leaves (eucalyptus), flowers and leaves (lavender), fruit (lemon), seeds (fennel), stem (lemongrass), wood (sandalwood), berries (juniper), root (ginger), bark (cinnamon) or flower bud (clove). One plant may produce different essential oils from different parts of its structure. For example an orange tree will give essential oil of orange from the fruit, oil of petitgrain from the leaves and oil of neroli from the blossoms.

Essential oil is present in tiny glands or sacs, either on the surface of the plant or deep within the cellular structure. Essential oils are obtained mainly by distillation, where the plant material is packed tightly into a container through which steam is passed. The essences, which are highly volatile, evaporate into the steam and are carried along with it. As the distillate cools the essential oil separates from the water and is collected. Oils from the citrus fruits of lemon, grapefruit, orange and bergamot are obtained by squeezing the rind of the fruit. This method is called 'expression'.

The amount of essence present in a plant varies from species to species and whereas 100 kilos of eucalyptus leaves can yield 10 litres of essential oil, the same weight of rose petals may yield only half a litre (about 30 roses per drop of essential oil). This is obviously reflected in the price of different oils, with rose (otto), true melissa and neroli being the most expensive. As well as essential oils, 'absolutes' and resins are also available. These have a different chemical structure, being obtained by a method involving solvents, and there is usually some solvent present in the end product. Jasmine oil is only available as an absolute.

■ Names of Essential Oils

The name of a particular essential oil on a label is often followed by the latin name and occasionally by the country or place of origin. On the label of the essential oil of sandalwood, one may find the word 'Mysore', which is the old name for the mountainous districts in Southern India where the trees grow which produce the best essential oil of sandalwood.

There are occasionally two or three essential oils from completely different plants, yet bearing the same common name, for example chamomile. There are three plants whose essential oils appear to have some therapeutic properties in common, and yet each has its own, individual therapeutic benefits. *German chamomile* (Matricaria chamomilla) has a high proportion of azulin, which gives it a dark blue colour and makes it a preferable choice when treating skin conditions. *Roman chamomile* (Anthemis nobilis) is a blue/green colour and is the most useful of the chamomiles. *Morrocan chamomile* (Ormenis mixta) is not a chamomile at all, although it has many of the properties of roman chamomile. As it is less expensive, it is a very useful substitute. Marjoram is another example. The oil most used is spanish marjoram which is derived from a species of thyme known as Thymus mastichina. This oil is less expensive but harsher than sweet marjoram, which comes from the plant Origanum majorana. Both oils share some similar properties, but each has its own benefits as well.

■ Purchasing Essential Oils

Unfortunately, essential oils are easily adulterated by the addition of alcohol, synthetics or cheaper essential oils, thus diluting their therapeutic properties. It is therefore important to buy oils from a reliable supplier who specialises in high quality essential oils. It should state on the bottle that the oils are pure and whether or not they have been diluted in a carrier. Some essential oils can be bought already diluted in carrier oil, although they may be sold in 10ml bottles making them appear to be pure essential oils.

Perfume and fragrance oils are also available, for example perfume oils of hyacinth, jasmine, rose and white musk. These are neither therapeutic nor essential oils and are largely synthetic, used only for their fragrance. Jasmine and rose *absolutes* are available, although if the price is not at least ten times that of lavender, they are likely to be fragrances of synthetic origin.

■ Storage

Essential oils should be stored in brown glass bottles in a cool, dark place, and in their undiluted state in fully filled bottles may last for several years. The bottles should not be left on open shelves near light or sun and the lids should always be replaced firmly, to prevent deterioration and the escape of the more volatile elements of the oil. Once an essential oil has been added to carrier oil to make a massage oil it will last for only 3 or 4 months. However, wheatgerm carrier oil is a natural preservative and if 5% of it is added to the general carrier oil, the massage oil should keep for a further couple of months before going rancid.

6

Popular Essential Oils

There are over one hundred essential oils generally available and the following chapter describes some of the more popular oils and their uses. The most exotic, luxurious and expensive oils have been omitted. Although wonderful to use, they fall outside the budgets of most people and certainly most Health, Education and Social Services Departments! These oils include neroli, rose otto, rose absolute, jasmine absolute, and true melissa.

The relaxing oils of bergamot, cedarwood, chamomile, clary sage, cypress, geranium, juniper, lavender, marjoram, sandalwood and ylang ylang are described, and where an oil is relaxing *and* uplifting this is indicated. The invigorating oils of eucalyptus, lemon, peppermint and rosemary are included, together with oil of tea tree, to complete a useful basic kit of essential oils. The Therapeutic Index at the end of Chapter 12, gives further specific information about which essential oils to use when treating many common, minor conditions.

■ Bergamot *(Citrus bergamia)*

Bergamot is a citrus fruit and the essential oil is extracted from the peel by expression. It has a light fresh fragrance and the oil comes mainly from Southern Italy. The essential oil of bergamot has both relaxing and refreshing properties. Earl Grey tea is made by impregnating tea leaves with bergamot oil and it is also known as one of the main ingredients in Eau de Cologne. As a result of its ability to increase the photosensitivity of the skin, it was widely used in sun preparations some years ago.

Caution: As bergamot oil makes the skin more sensitive to light, it should never be used prior to exposure to natural or artificial sunlight.

Bergamot is indicated for the following conditions:

Digestive:	*appetite loss, flatulence, gastro-enteritis, indigestion*
Emotional:	*anxiety, depression*
Excretory:	*cystitis, urinary infections*
General:	*body and breath odour, earache*
Skin:	*acne, dermatitis, eczema, herpes (use with care), oiliness, ulcers, wounds*

■ Cedarwood *(Cedrus atlantica)*

The best cedarwood for medicinal purposes comes from the tree Cedrus atlantica and was one of the oils used in the preservation of Egyptian mummies. It has a woody odour which some people find reminiscent of sharpening pencils at school, as cedarwood is one of the main woods used for making pencils. The wood is comminuted (chopped into small pieces) and then distilled to obtain the oil.

Cedarwood is a relaxing essential oil and can have a considerable effect on chronic anxiety. It is helpful in respiratory problems which involve catarrh, including coughs and bronchitis. Cystitis is another condition helped by cedarwood and it is useful against dandruff and in the control of an oily skin and scalp.

Cedarwood, useful as an insect repellent, is indicated for the following conditions:

Emotional:	*anxiety*
Excretory:	*cystitis*
Respiratory:	*bronchitis, catarrh, coughs*
Skin:	*acne, alopecia, dandruff, irritated skin, seborrhoea of the scalp*

■ Chamomile *(Anthemis nobilis)*

The little yellow daisy-like flowers together with the leaves are used in the distillation of roman chamomile. It is grown in Europe and England and, like lavender, the oil is very versatile.

This soothing and relaxing essential oil is excellent for the nervous system, helping sufferers of insomnia and irritability as well as stress. It is an uplifting oil which can be used for depression. Well known for its healing effects on many skin disorders, it can also help digestive and muscular problems (including most forms of arthritis).

Roman chamomile is indicated for the following conditions:

Digestive:	*appetite loss, constipation, indigestion, nausea*
Emotional:	*anxiety, depression, irritability*
General:	*conjunctivitis, earache, insomnia, headaches*
Muscular:	*aches, pains, rheumatism, rheumatoid arthritis, cramp*
Reproductive:	*heavy periods, irregular periods, menopause, painful periods, pre-menstrual tension*
Skin:	*acne, allergies, broken veins, dermatitis, dryness, eczema, inflammation, irritation, sensitivity*

■ Clary Sage *(Salvia sclarea)*

This beautiful plant grows high in the pre-Alps and the plant is 4 - 5 feet high with branches of plump florets in varying shades of mauve/ pink growing on a central stem. One single stem of clary sage in a vase will fill a large room with its warm nutty aroma.

The oil, taken from the whole flowering top, is extremely useful for menstrual problems and has relaxing and uplifting properties. Clary sage water makes an excellent skin tonic for the mature or inflamed skin.

Clary sage is indicated for the following conditions:

Circulatory:	*high blood pressure*
Emotional:	*anxiety, depression,*
Reproductive:	*irregular periods, pre-menstrual tension, painful periods*
Skin:	*inflammation, maturity, sensitivity*

■ Cypress *(Cupressus sempervirens)*

Cypress is a relaxing, soothing oil which can reduce stress and irritability. The essential oil is distilled from the leaves and twigs of cypress trees grown in Germany and France.

One of its main benefits is its stimulatory effect on the circulatory system. It is excellent for varicose veins, broken capillaries and haemorrhoids. It is also helpful for several menstrual disorders, including the menopause and some ovary problems.

This relaxing yet tonic essential oil is indicated for the following conditions:

Circulatory:	*poor circulation, haemorrhoids, varicose veins*
Digestive:	*diarrhoea*
Emotional:	*anxiety, irritability*
Excretory:	*haemorrhoids, fluid retention*
General:	*nose bleeds*
Reproductive:	*heavy menopausal bleeding, painful periods*
Muscular:	*cramp*
Respiratory:	*asthma, coughs*
Skin:	*broken veins, maturity, oiliness*

■ Eucalyptus *(Eucalyptus globulus)*

Although the eucalyptus tree is one of the largest in the world those grown for their essential oil are pruned each year to keep the leaves within easy reach for picking. There are over three hundred varieties of eucalyptus and most of the oil used to come from Australia.

Production is now much higher in Spain, Portugal, Africa and China. The oil is situated inside the leaf structure and the leaf needs to be broken to release the aroma.

Eucalyptus is most effective when used for respiratory conditions, from the simple blocked nose to chronic coughing and bronchial asthma. It is also used effectively to relieve muscular ailments and to strengthen the kidneys.

Eucalyptus is useful as an insect repellent and is indicated for the following conditions:

Excretory:	*cystitis, fluid retention, urinary infections*
General:	*congestive headache*
Muscular:	*aches, pains, rheumatism, rheumatoid arthritis*
Respiratory:	*asthma, bronchitis, catarrh, head colds, coughs, sinusitis*
Skin:	*herpes simplex, ulcers, wounds*

■ Geranium *(Pelargonium odoratissimum)*

Essential oil of geranium has a sweet, fresh floral scent and is well known for its relaxing and uplifting properties. The highest quality geranium used to come from the Bourbon Islands, but some geranium oil from France has a comparable aroma. Egyptian and Chinese oils are less expensive and the aroma is a little sharper.

Geranium has cleansing and healing effects on the skin and is useful also for menstrual disorders, obesity and certain excretory and digestive disorders.

Geranium is indicated for the following conditions:

Digestive:	*diabetes, diarrhoea, gastro-enteritis*
Emotional:	*anxiety, depression*
Excretory:	*fluid retention, urinary infection*
Reproductive:	*menopausal bleeding, pre-menstrual tension*
Skin:	*cellulite, dryness, inflammation, eczema, dermatitis, oiliness*

■ Juniper *(Juniperus communis)*

The best quality juniper oil is distilled only from the fruits of the juniper bush and is sold as juniperberry oil. All other juniper oils are distilled from leaves, twigs and berries and the poorest quality is distilled using berries which have already had some properties extracted from them for making gin. The oil is extracted from trees grown in various parts of the world, mainly France and Canada.

One of its main uses is with the excretory system. It is a good detoxifier and as such is very useful in dealing with urinary disorders and fluid retention. Juniper is excellent for relieving muscular aches and pains and helping many forms of arthritis. It is also helpful to the nervous system, being both a tonic and a sedative, and able to promote sleep in those whose minds are continuously in a worried state.

Juniper is indicated for the following conditions:

Circulatory:	*poor circulation*
Digestive:	*diabetes, flatulence, indigestion*
Emotional:	*anxiety, insomnia*
Excretory:	*cystitis, fluid retention, urinary infection*
Muscular:	*aches, pains, rheumatism, rheumatoid arthritis*
Reproductive:	*infrequent menstruation, irregular periods, painful periods*
Skin:	*acne, cellulite, dermatitis, eczema, oiliness (also scalp)*

■ Lavender *(Lavendula officinalis)*

Lavender is the best loved and universally popular oil, often referred to as the 'essential essential oil'. It is difficult to obtain a genuine unadulterated lavender. The best lavender comes from France, though a good quality oil can be obtained from Bulgaria and Yugoslavia. Lavender is frequently adulterated through the use of lavandin. Lavandin is a very hardy plant, a hybrid of lavender and rich in essential oil. The aroma is not as sweet although it is believed by some to have quite a few of the therapeutic properties of lavender. It is a simple matter to add synthetic lavender aroma to lavandin when the demand for lavender is higher than production, and this results in an oil with much fewer therapeutic properties than true lavender, or indeed true *lavandin.*

Lavender has a healing effect on disorders of practically every system of the body. Its most renowned attributes are its ability to promote rapid healing, and the pain relieving ability of the oil when used, for example, immediately after a burn. It is helpful for stress, depression, headaches and insomnia; it both relaxes and tones muscles, is beneficial in many respiratory disorders and of course is a great healer for skin problems of many kinds.

Lavender is indicated in the following conditions:

Circulatory:	*high blood pressure*
Digestive:	*diarrhoea, flatulence, gastro-enteritis, indigestion, nausea*
Emotional:	*anxiety, depression, insomnia, irritability, palpitations*
Excretory:	*fluid retention*
General:	*burns, earache, headaches, migraine, scars, wounds*
Muscular:	*aches, pains, rheumatism, sprains*
Reproductive:	*infrequent menstruation, irregular periods, painful periods, pre-menstrual tension*
Respiratory:	*asthma, coughs, sinusitis, sore throat*
Skin:	*acne, cellulite, dermatitis, eczema, dryness, inflammation, oiliness, sensitivity, stretch marks*

■ Lemon *(Citrus limonum)*

Lemon and other citrus fruit oils are not obtained by distillation but by expression. The oil glands are in the zest and are extracted now mostly by mechanical means after the juice has been removed. The dual use of citrus fruits keeps these oils at a reasonable price. Essential oil of lemon is produced in Sicily, Cyprus and Italy and it takes 3 kilos of lemons to produce one kilo of essential oil. Lemon has far more attributes than was at first thought, which may be true for many essential oils. It invigorates the mind and is also beneficial for circulatory disorders including high blood pressure, anaemia and varicose veins. Essential oil of lemon has also been found to be useful in muscular and respiratory disorders.

Caution: Do not use more than 2 drops of lemon oil in a bath if the person's skin is very sensitive.

Lemon is indicated for the following conditions:

Circulatory:	*high blood pressure, poor circulation, varicose veins*
Digestive:	*appetite loss, diabetes, diarrhoea*
General:	*boils, insect bites, mouth ulcers, verrucas*
Muscular:	*aches, pains, rheumatism, rheumatoid arthritis*
Respiratory:	*asthma, 'flu, head colds*
Skin:	*broken veins, herpes simplex, maturity, oiliness*

■ Marjoram *(Origanum majorana)*

Marjoram oil is relaxing, and is the most sedative of all essential oils. The oil comes from the flowering heads of the sweet marjoram grown in Southern France, Spain and Tunisia. It is helpful in situations where a person is irritable, has insomnia, or suffers from pre-menstrual tension which may be stress related. This oil is also used widely in muscular disorders including cramp, sprains, bruises and rheumatism (see reference to marjoram on page 33).

Marjoram is indicated for the following conditions:

Circulatory:	*high blood pressure*
Digestive:	*constipation, stomach cramp*
Emotional:	*anxiety, insomnia, irritability*
General:	*headaches, migraine*
Muscular:	*aches, pains, bruises, cramp, rheumatism, rheumatoid arthritis*
Reproductive:	*painful periods, pre-menstrual tension*
Respiratory:	*asthma, catarrh*

■ Peppermint *(Mentha piperita)*

English peppermint is reputed to be of the best quality although, together with French peppermint, it is more costly than the American oil, which has a sharper aroma. The best oil is distilled from the dark green leaves and flowering tops of the Mitcham mint and is widely used in the toiletries and food industry.

It is carminative (expels flatulence) to the digestive system. It also invigorates the mind and improves concentration.

Caution: Do not use more than 2 drops of peppermint in a bath if the skin is sensitive.

Peppermint is useful as an insect repellent and is indicated for the following conditions :

Digestive:	*diarrhoea, flatulence, indigestion, nausea, travel sickness*
Emotional:	*general debility, shock*
General:	*headaches and migraines (digestive origin)*
Reproductive:	*infrequent menstruation, irregular periods, painful periods*
Respiratory:	*asthma, bronchitis, catarrh, coughs, 'flu, head colds*
Skin:	*inflammation, irritation*

■ Rosemary *(Rosamarinus officinalis)*

Rosemary is distilled from the wonderfully aromatic leaves of the plant, and the best oil comes from Southern France, although rosemary is also grown in Morocco, Tunisia and Spain. The quality and aroma varies and it is an easy oil to adulterate.

It is an oil well known for its normalising effect on the digestive system, being particularly helpful in cases of constipation. It is a warm stimulating oil which is used for its uplifting and refreshing effects on the mind. Rosemary is a stimulant of both the lymph and the blood circulatory systems, and disorders giving muscular pain can be effectively relieved by its use. Other attributes include its cleansing effects on the skin, making it extremely useful for dandruff and wounds.

Rosemary is indicated for the following conditions :

Circulatory:	*poor circulation (also lymph)*
Digestive:	*constipation, flatulence, gastro-enteritis, stomach pains*
Emotional:	*general debility, mental fatigue*
Excretory:	*fluid retention*
General:	*headaches, migraines, wounds*
Muscular:	*aches, pains, rheumatism, rheumatoid arthritis*
Reproductive:	*infrequent menstruation*
Respiratory:	*asthma, bronchitis, coughs, 'flu, head colds*
Skin:	*alopecia, dandruff, scalp disorders*

■ Sandalwood *(Santalum album)*

The sandalwood tree takes thirty years to reach maturity. As the heartwood takes three years to reach seven centimetres in diameter and this is the main part of the tree distilled for its essential oil, sandalwood oil is naturally quite costly. The highest quality sandalwood comes from what used to be called Mysore in India and has a sweet, woody, oriental aroma.

It has excellent relaxing properties and is also very useful for respiratory disorders involving catarrh or irritated mucus membranes as in a sore throat. It can help certain digestive complaints and is a favourite choice for a dry, irritable or inflamed skin.

Sandalwood is indicated for the following conditions:

Digestive:	*diarrhoea, gastro-enteritis, nausea*
Emotional:	*anxiety, depression*
Excretory:	*cystitis, urinary infections*
Respiratory:	*bronchitis, catarrh, sore throat*
Skin:	*dryness, inflamation, irritation*

■ Tea Tree *(Melaleuca alternifolia)*

The Tea Tree is native to Australia, where the aborigines have used it medicinally for centuries. Recently, the Australian Government invested in wholesale production of this useful tree, and the many resulting plantations are now responsible for the whole world's supply of the oil.

Tea tree has powerful bactericidal properties and is many times more powerful in this respect than phenol, which of course cannot be put on the skin. Tea tree, amazingly, is very kind to the skin, which makes it useful for the treatment of spots and acne, and as a gargle against winter infections.

Tea tree is indicated for the following conditions :

Digestive:	*indigestion, candida albicans, gastro-enteritis*
General:	*mouth infections (eg. thrush), insect bites*
Reproductive:	*vaginal thrush*
Respiratory:	*bronchitis, coughs, head colds, sore throat*
Skin:	*acne*

■ Ylang Ylang *(Cananga odorata)*

This exotic plant is grown mainly in the Phillipines and Reunion. The tree flowers all the year round, but the best essential oil is produced from blossoms picked in May and June. From the distillation process, which is complicated, three or four qualities of ylang ylang are produced. It has a sweet, heady fragrance and is sometimes known as 'poor man's jasmine'.

Ylang Ylang is indicated for the following conditions :

Circulatory:	*high blood pressure*
Digestive:	*gastro-enteritis*
Emotional:	*anxiety, depression, insomnia*
Skin:	*oiliness*

7

Carriers of Essential Oils

Essential oils are used by diluting them in a carrier, which is anything which carries the essential oil into the body. The main carriers are air, water and massage oil or lotion. Pure undiluted essential oils should not be used directly on the skin as they are extremely concentrated and could cause irritation. There are a few exceptions to this as a few drops of lavender or tea tree essential oil may be used as an emergency measure on spots, burns, stings or small cuts.

■ Air as a Carrier

There are two main ways in which air can be used as a carrier, either through inhalation or by using a vaporiser, which, through heat, enables the essential oil to evaporate more quickly into the atmosphere.

Inhalation is probably the most important and certainly the quickest way in which essential oils enter the body. The oils reach the brain via the cilia at the top of the nose which have direct access to the brain through the olfactory nerves. All other access to the brain has to be made through the blood-brain barrier, which is not as easily penetrated, being designed to keep out harmful substances which may be in the food we eat.

Emotional conditions such as stress, and physical problems such as respiratory disorders can be helped by using inhalation or the vaporisation of particular essential oils.

Inhalation

This method is particularly suited to relieving stress and treating physical ailments such as sinus problems, colds and flu, breathing difficulties and congestion.

Similar methods have been used for years. For example, a mother rubbing Vick onto her child's chest when she has a cold is in fact using a mixture of oils of eucalyptus, nutmeg, cedarwood and camphor to help relieve the congestion. The practice of putting eucalyptus oil on the coals of a sauna is designed to have the same effect.

There are three main ways of helping a person to inhale essential oils directly: by placing drops on a handkerchief, by putting a few drops on the pillow or by using a bowl of water.

Inhalation Using Essential Oil on a Handkerchief

This method simply involves placing between 2 and 6 drops of essential oil on a person's handkerchief and encouraging her to hold it regularly to her nose and inhale deeply. Essential oils of eucalyptus or peppermint are common oils to be used in this way (see Therapeutic Index).

Caution: If the person has a tendency to rub her handkerchief near her eye then use this method with caution as essential oils will irritate the eyes and could make them smart. Placing a tissue with oils in her blouse or using the oils in a vaporiser may be better alternatives.

Inhalation Using Essential Oils on the Pillow

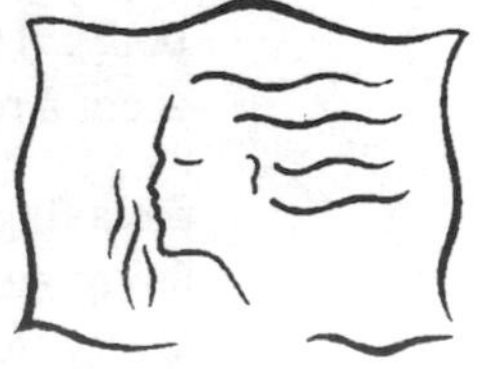

To help ease a person's breathing during the night, 6 to 8 drops of essential oil could be placed on a handkerchief or cotton wool ball inside the pillow slip. Some writers recommend putting essential oils directly onto the pillow; however this could irritate the skin if the cheek lies directly onto it, and may also stain the pillow. 'Pillow Pets' could be made for young children. These might be made into the shape of any favourite animal with a space inside to place a handkerchief fragranced with essential oils.

Inhalation Over a Bowl of Hot Water

This method involves using a bowl of very hot (but not boiling) water into which 2 to 6 drops of essential oil are placed. The person should then lean over the bowl for 1 to 3 minutes, closing her eyes and

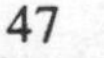

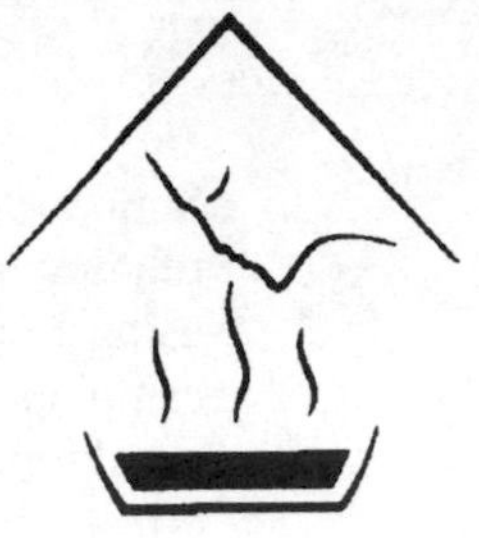

placing a towel over the head to ensure that the vapour does not disappear too quickly. Alternatively a facial sauna can be used.

Inhaling essential oils in this way for several minutes can ease breathing, and one of the most effective essential oils to choose is eucalyptus, either singly or in combination with other essential oils.

Caution: This method should not be used if a person suffers from asthma, as the steam *may* aggravate rather than alleviate breathing difficulties. However, people who have asthma can use essential oils on a handkerchief or in the bath. In the latter the drops are dispersed over a greater area and their vapour is less concentrated.

Obviously using a bowl requires not only co-operation from the person with a learning difficulty but also an awareness of safety precautions when using hot water. For individuals who have severe learning difficulties the following method may be a better alternative.

Vaporisation

Here water is used, usually together with heat, to enable the oils to vaporise more quickly into the air, which then carries them into the body. There are many ways of vaporising essential oils either just to scent a room or to create a specific atmosphere.

Relaxing oils could be used to create a soothing, calming atmosphere. Invigorating, uplifting oils can be used to create a more energetic and lively 'feel'. If breathing is a problem, oils which are helpful for breathing difficulties can be vaporised (see Therapeutic Index).

This method is a particularly useful way of decreasing the possibilty of infection, as all essential oils are antiseptic. Some of them (e.g. tea tree) are stronger than phenol (carbolic acid).

There are several ways of vaporising essential oils: by using a burner, vaporising ring, bowl of hot water, saucer of water or ball of cotton wool on a radiator, or in an air spray. In all of these methods up to 12 drops of essential oils can be used depending on the strength of fragrance required. Essential oils can be used singly, although if up to 4 different oils are used, the effect is enhanced, due to the synergistic nature of essential oils. For example 4 drops each of essential oil of lavender, geranium and bergamot produces a particularly pleasant and relaxing aroma.

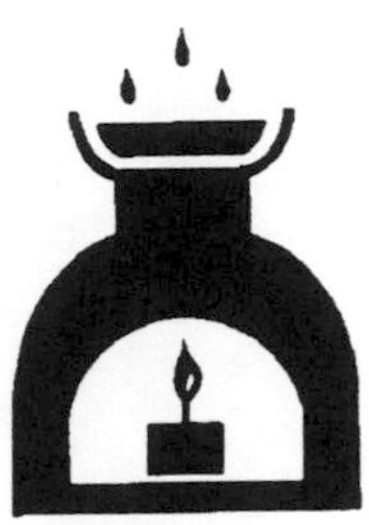

Essential Oil Burners

There are many different types of burners available, from simple terracotta to more elaborate and expensive ceramic vaporisers and burners. Electric diffusers are also available.

Each burner has a saucer which is either detachable or attached to the main body of the burner. Underneath the saucer of a non-electric burner a night light candle is placed. The saucer should be half filled with water into which 6 to 12 drops of essential oil are placed. The candle is then lit to produce the heat which vaporises the oil in the saucer. The water and oils can be topped up as they evaporate. Always keep an eye on the water level and *do not* allow it to burn dry.

For safety reasons non-electric burners may not be suitable in certain situations. If a burner is intended for use in a Sensory or Snoezelen type room it is important that the Health and Safety Officer is aware of this. A small fire extinguisher similar to those kept in cars should be made available if this method is to be used in a school or day centre. Electric vaporisers and diffusers are the safest to use.

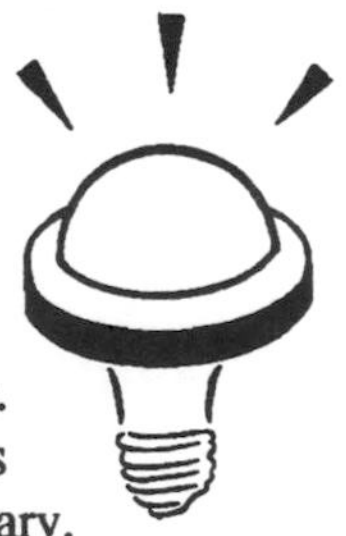

Vaporising Rings

A vaporising ring is a small metal or ceramic ring which fits neatly onto the light bulb in a lamp. The ring can be half filled with water to which essential oils are added or essential oils can be added directly into the ring. When the lamp is switched on, the fragrance of the oils is released. Water and oil need to be replaced when necessary. This method provides an unobtrusive and safe way of scenting a room with the minimum of effort. Use only low power bulbs (below 100 watts).

Vaporisation Using Water

Where the above methods are not possible, essential oils can be vaporised simply by using either a small bowl or a saucer of water. A bowl of hot water containing essential oils can be used or, more simply, a saucer of water to which essential oils are added can be placed on a radiator, or next to a fan heater.

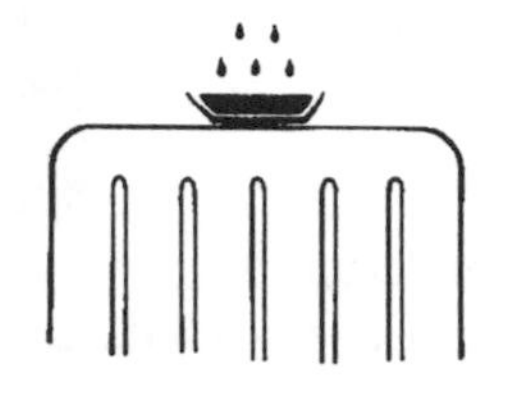

Another alternative is to put 6-8 drops of essential oil onto a ball of cotton wool, or a kitchen tissue, and place this next to the pipe of a radiator.

Airspray

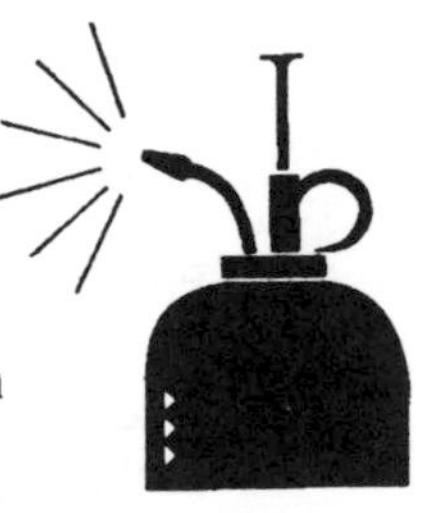

Essential oils can be added to the atmosphere by dispersing them first in water and then spraying them into the air. House plant sprayers are useful for this, with 20 drops added to half a pint of water to fragrance a room or to protect against infection. Up to 40 drops can be used if a stronger effect is required. Ceramic sprayers are best as the essential oil does not react with pottery. However, plastic sprayers can be used providing that any unused water is discarded and the sprayer is washed after use.

N.B. As only 20% of an essential oil dissolves in water, the sprayer needs to be shaken vigorously before spraying.

■ Water as a carrier

Water is used as the carrier in baths and compresses. Although it is slower than inhalation as a method of carrying essential oils into the body, research has shown that twenty minutes after a person has had a bath with 4 drops of lavender in the water, evidence of the oil can be found in the person's urine.

N.B. As some medication can make a person's skin sensitive, no more than 6 drops of oil should be used in baths and compresses.

Aromatic Baths

Aromatic baths can be used to relax, to invigorate or to help certain disorders including aches and pains, urinary infections, insomnia, arthritis, etc.

For maximum effectiveness run a warm bath and add 4 to 6 drops of essential oil *after the bath has been run* (use only 4 drops if the skin is ultra sensitive). If you add essential oil whilst the water is running, some of the more volatile elements will evaporate before the person gets in. Disperse the oil well by agitating the water and then encourage the person to stay in the water for ten to fifteen minutes.

For those who prefer bubbles in the bath, essential oils can be added to a tablespoon of foaming bath oil before being added to the water. If the person has a particularly dry skin, the essential oils can be added to a teaspoonful of vegetable oil before being put in the bath. The same quantities of essential oils (4 to 6 drops) can be used in all these methods. The effects of the oils are subtle and can be perceived up to a couple of hours after the bath.

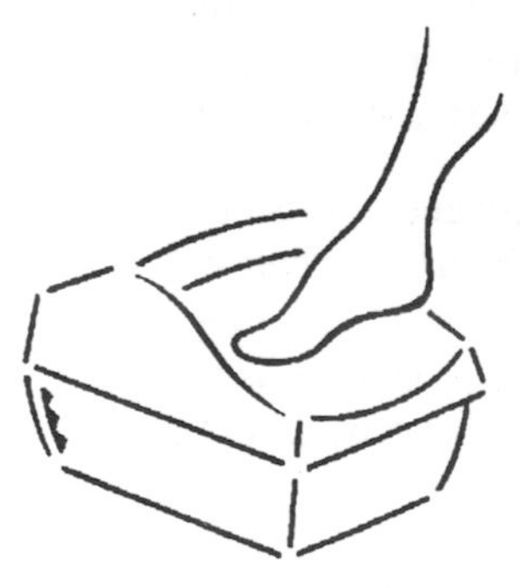

Foot baths, used to warm or relax the feet, would be enhanced by the addition of relevant essential oils. Foot baths could also be used to treat athletes foot or improve the circulation. If used as part of a sensory awareness or stimulation session at school, then essential oils in a foot spa could provide olfactory stimulation in addition to vibration and touch. During a relaxation session at a school, day centre or at home, 4 to 6 drops of essential oil would be needed using, for example, lavender, ylang ylang and sandalwood.

Caution: Children under 10 years should only have 2 to 4 drops of essential oil added to their bath (children under two and babies, only 1 - 2 drops). The drops should be diluted in a teaspoon of carrier oil, full fat milk, cream or honey before being added to the water. For people with sensitive skin only two drops of lemon, peppermint, lemongrass, basil, thyme or fennel should be used, making it up to the number of drops needed with any other essential oils listed.

Compresses

A compress can be used to treat small wounds, to draw out bruising or strains or to help to alleviate earache, ulcers and varicose veins. 2 to 6 drops of the relevant essential oil (see Therapeutic Index) are added to *just* enough water to soak into the cotton material needed for the affected area.

Cold compresses are useful for migraine and headaches, perhaps using 2 drops of peppermint and 2 drops of lavender in the water and applying the compress to the brow or the back of the neck. Hot compresses can be used for muscular pain or period pains. Compresses using essential oils can be used immediately after an accident before taking the person to a G.P. or hospital. They can also be used to treat more long term conditions including ulcers and varicose veins.

■ Massage Oils and Lotions as Carriers

Massage is an excellent way of introducing essential oils into the body since they readily dissolve in vegetable oil, which acts as the lubricant and carries them evenly over the skin for penetration. The qualities which are required for a good base carrier oil are that it is odourless and has a light consistency and a smooth texture.

Carrier oils, unlike essential oils, are greasy and nourish the skin. There are many vegetable oils which can be used as carriers. Mineral oils such as baby oil are not recommended as they can clog the skin's pores and do not have the same penetrative properties as vegetable oils. In addition mineral oils, unlike vegetable oils, do not add vitamins to the skin.

There are general base carrier oils such as grapeseed, almond and safflower and more specialised carrier oils such as avocado and wheatgerm, which are thicker and more expensive. These last can be added to the base carrier oil (in proportions of 5% to 25%) as they are too heavy to be used on their own in massage. More than one specialised carrier oil can be added to a base carrier oil.

Always try to obtain an unrefined, cold-pressed oil (preferably first or virgin pressing) as the oil will be penetrating the skin and therefore needs to be of high quality. Organically grown vegetable oils are rare but are obviously good to use. Carrier oils can usually be purchased at good health food shops or mail-order from companies which supply essential oils and carrier oils to aromatherapists.

Other specialised carrier oils include calendula, jojoba, St. John's wort and evening primrose.

N.B. Carrier oils which are marked "pure" and are sold for cooking are usually of an inferior quality and are steam extracted, bleached and deodorised with chemicals.

Wheatgerm oil is rich in Vitamin E and being an excellent anti-oxidant it helps to extend the life of the massage oil (once essential oils are added). If it is not used the massage oil would soon become rancid and may become cloudy.

Avocado oil has excellent penetrative properties so that when added to a base carrier oil it can help the essential oils penetrate the skin more quickly.

For people who prefer a non-oily medium, an emulsified *vegetable*, non-perfumed carrier lotion can be used. It penetrates the skin quickly leaving a non-oily feel to the skin. Although it is not suitable for long massage sequences, it is ideal for a short hand, foot or facial massage or for self application.

Making Up a Massage Oil or Lotion

The general principle for making up a massage oil or lotion is to use 1 to 2 drops of essential oil for every 5ml (one teaspoon) of carrier oil or lotion. To make up 50ml of massage oil put 15-20 drops of essential oil into a clean 50ml bottle (available from a pharmacy) and top up with a base carrier oil such as grapeseed. These 15-20 drops can be made up of three or four different oils. When adding essential oils to a carrier lotion the same principle applies. However, it is easier to add the essential oils to 75% of the lotion, giving plenty of air space for mixing in the oils thoroughly. The remaining 25% can then be added and the bottle reshaken.

To make a massage oil which has good penetrative properties and will not go rancid quickly, avocado and wheatgerm should be added. Put 15 - 20 drops of essential oil into a bottle and add one teaspoon of avocado oil and one teaspoon of wheatgerm oil. Top up to 50ml with grapeseed oil as before.

There is no need to add wheatgerm when preparing a massage lotion as the latter's keeping qualities are far in excess of that of a vegetable oil. When making a massage oil for children under 10 years old or adults over 75, use half the number of drops used for an adult, i.e. 8 to 10 drops in 50ml of carrier oil. The children's recipe is also suitable for babies, since the area being covered with oil decreases with age and, therefore, less oil is applied.

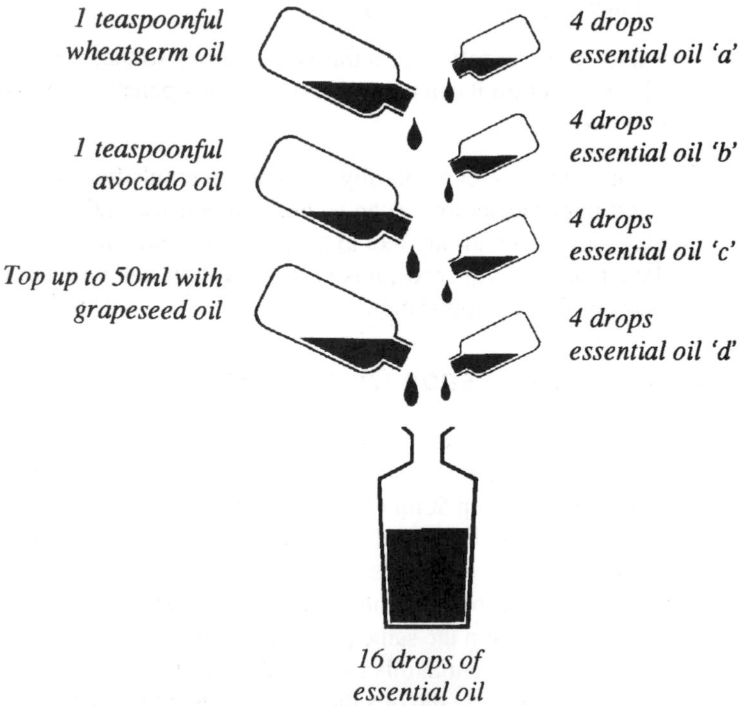

Summary of the Different Ways of Using Essential Oils

Air as a Carrier

Inhalation using essential oils

1. On a handkerchief
2. Inside a pillow slip
3. In a bowl of hot water (inhaling directly)

Vaporisation of essential oils

1. In a burner
2. In a vaporising ring
3. In a bowl of hot water (inhaling indirectly)
4. In a saucer of water or on a cotton wool ball (or tissue) on a radiator
5. In an airspray

Water as a Carrier

1. In the bath
2. On a compress

Oil or Lotion as a Carrier

1. In a massage oil or lotion

8

Aromatherapy and Massage to Relax

Aromatherapy is perhaps best known as a most effective way of relaxing. Massage, on its own, relaxes the mind and body, countering the negative effects of everyday stresses. When combined with the properties of the relaxing essential oils the effects are even more soothing and calming, and they last much longer. Books and self help courses suggest that many illnesses and diseases are either directly linked to, or aggravated by, a person's inability to cope with stress. These include skin conditions, digestive complaints, pre-menstrual tension, migraine, headaches, insomnia, high blood pressure, heart attacks, asthma and arthritis. Stress and illness appear to be closely related.

Stress is not exclusive to the high powered business person but can occur whenever there is a challenge or confrontation. People who have learning difficulties regularly experience the extreme frustration of not being listened to and having very little control over their lives. As the situation begins to change, these people encounter new, positive challenges of speaking up in advocacy groups, in individual personal planning meetings and in other situations which although very positive may also be stressful. This is not to suggest that these opportunities should not be sought and encouraged, but to acknowledge that support in dealing with confrontation and stress is also required.

■ Relaxation to Help to Reduce Challenging Behaviours

Some challenging behaviours are often the only way that a person can clearly express distress, anger, frustration or grief. Often disruptive behaviour is precipitated by tension and anxiety (Bijou, 1966. Peck, 1977. Zigler, 1966). It may be the only choice that a person has available to her to make her needs or feelings known.

It is interesting to look at the choices which babies make in order to get their needs met, as they illustrate in a simple form principles which are exactly the same when people become older and life becomes more complex. If a baby has hunger sensations she has a number of options: to wake and cry; to wake and scream; to wake and ignore the hunger sensations because she knows they will soon be met; to wake and make sounds indicative of discomfort or to find something else of more interest.

However, the different options have different consequences. Screaming may get the quickest results but may also bring a tired, bad-tempered parent and inadequate food supply. Waking and waiting may lead to even more discomfort. A combination of the baby's own choice and the way that the expression is met will condition the way that the baby chooses to react. In future similar situations the baby will go for one option rather than another. The crucial part of this is the response that the baby's choice of expression receives. The more a person's power or ability to choose is acknowledged and respected, the greater the possibilities for healthy development of choice-making (Oliver, L. 1987).

One of the challenges and responsibilities of working with people, particularly those who have severe or profound learning difficulties, is to help each person to find appropriate ways of expressing and communicating their needs, feelings and desires, and tuning into and recognising distressed or stuck patterns of behaviours which are inappropriate or no longer useful for the person to have. Challenging behaviours such as screaming, withdrawal or some forms of self-injury may well be the only way a person has found to communicate how she is feeling when she is unable to say;

I'm frightened
I don't like it here
I don't want to do this
I don't feel well
I am angry
I am tired
I feel bored
I don't like the way you touch me

Aromatherapy and massage do not provide miracle answers. They can become part of the solution, helping the person to feel reassured, supported and recognised by another person. Massage can also help a person to become more aware of her body's state, identifying when muscles are tight and enjoying the feeling of complete relaxation which massage with essential oils can bring.

Relaxation has been shown to be successful in the treatment of psychomotor seizures (Wells et al, 1978), self-injurious behaviour (Steen and Zuriff, 1977), and phobias (Peck, 1977) in people who have learning difficulties.

In 1989 McPhail and Chamore published results of research, to assess the effects of relaxation training on subsequent disruptive behaviour with two groups of six adults with learning difficulties and verbal, aggressive, movement or other disruptive behaviour.

> The results clearly showed that...relaxation significantly and substantially reduces disruptive behaviour in mentally handicapped adults. All four categories of behaviour measured were reduced by relaxation, and two of them (verbal and aggression) were significantly different from the control group. The greatest decrease was for aggression and the other disruptive behaviours which were eliminated for the rest of the day...Unlike that found in the other studies where training sessions were infrequent, the effects of daily training in relaxation in this study were immediate and also cumulative.

Significantly, as no attempt was made to teach relaxation as a coping skill, three months later the disruptive behaviour had returned. It would be interesting to extend this study and teach relaxation as a coping strategy.

Theory into Practice

John lives in a hospital for people who have learning difficulties. He is described as having challenging behaviour and he spends much of his time crawling on his hands and knees, often banging his head on the tiled floor. The hospital staff said that when they intervened and tried to stop this behaviour it appeared to make matters worse and John accelerated the behaviour. In the end the staff attempted to ignore the behaviour in the hope that he would 'work through it'.

When the aromatherapist met John he was rhythmically hitting his forehead on the floor and had sores and blood on his head. The aromatherapist used a relaxing blend of essential oils and began by introducing the aroma near to his face for him to smell. The aromatherapist talked as she began to massage his back using large circular strokes. John's response was positive and immediate and she began to use slightly firmer strokes. John straightened up and stopped banging his head as soon as the massage began. He sat on his knees, apparently fully absorbed, whilst his back was massaged for ten minutes. John remained peaceful for the rest of the afternoon.

It is important to remember that there may be physiological or other reasons for some challenging behaviours. People with Cornelia de Lange syndrome, for example, have a tendency towards self injurious behaviour. Favell, McGimsey and Schell (1982) indicate that from the results of their research, sensory reinforcement was the underlying reason for certain self-stimulatory and self-injurious acts. By providing alternative activities which stimulated the same senses, this behaviour abated.

Recent research also suggests that one reason for some self injurious behaviour could be that it stimulates the production of endorphines (Sandman et al 1983). Endorphines are the brain's natural opiates or pain blockers and can be 20-30 times more potent than the analgesic morphine. They are created inside the brain and are triggered by stimuli as diverse as pain, eating, sex, exercise, fear, music and meditation. In this way eating is comforting, and vigorous exercise leads to a 'runner's high'. The effect wears off within minutes. Massage also results in the production of endorphines and so could be a more appropriate way of introducing the same effect for someone who injures herself.

■ The Relaxing Properties of Essential Oils

Professor Paolo Rovesti, Director of the Instituto Derivati Vegetali in Milan, Italy, has conducted many clinical trials on the effectiveness of essential oils in dealing with anxiety and tension.

He states that:

> According to sociologists and neurologists the salient characteristics of our age are those of anxiety and depression, and the material proof of this is available in the even higher figures shown for the consumption of tranquillizers and stimulants...essential oils in the appropriate doses are harmless to the organism and do not cause trouble like those produced by ordinary psychological drugs. Very conclusive experiments in this direction have been carried out in various clinics for nervous diseases [1].

Aromatherapy and massage can be included with counselling and other measures for alleviating anxiety.

Many of the relaxing essential oils are also anti-depressant and without any of the unpleasant side effects associated with anti-depressant drugs.

Essential oils which are both relaxing and uplifting include:

Bergamot
Chamomile
Clary sage
Geranium
Lavender
Sandalwood
Ylang ylang

Other essential oils which promote relaxation include:

Cedarwood
Cypress
Juniper
Marjoram

Some essential oils have been shown to be effective in the treatment of insomnia and these include:

Chamomile
Juniper
Lavender
Marjoram
Sandalwood
Ylang ylang

By using these more sedative essential oils some nurses have found that the need for drugs to treat insomnia has been considerably reduced and in some cases no longer needed at all. One Sister working on a ward for elderly people said, "We began to use

1. Rovesti, P. 1971

essential oils to enhance the effect of massage, and discovered that we were able to reduce conventional drugs to a minimum. A bath with essential oils followed by a massage, plus a few drops on the pillow induced peaceful sleep'' (Passant, H. 1990).

At the Oxford Nursing Development Unit patients are offered an aromatherapy massage instead of analgesics or sedatives. The most commonly used sedative is a drug called Temazepam which now has a rival in terms of effectiveness on that ward in the form of marjoram and lavender.

■ Using Relaxing Essential Oils and Massage with People who have Learning Difficulties.

The following techniques could be used at home, as part of a relaxation session or as part of a health care session in a school or centre. They could be used to relax someone in preparation for another activity, to welcome a new person into a group or to make contact and reduce someone's anxiety or distress. Or find your own application...

1. Vaporising Relaxing Essential Oils

One way to use relaxing essential oils is to vaporise them using either a burner, vaporising ring or saucer of water on a radiator. They could be vaporised either singly or in combination to give a soothing and relaxing ambience. This may be particularly useful during relaxation sessions in a day centre or school, whilst people relax after work or generally during the evening before going to bed.

The research conducted at Warwick University (described in Chapter 2) suggests that a relaxing essential oil, for example lavender, could be vaporised regularly during a massage where the person feels calm and relaxed. Vaporising the same oil of lavender in situations where the person appears tense, could then have the effect of calming and relaxing her because of the unconscious association of that particular aroma.

2. Using Relaxing Oils in the Bath

A good night's sleep can be induced by using a few drops of a relaxing essential oil in the bath before going to bed. Any of the relaxing oils could be chosen depending on the person's favourite, concentrating on the more sedative oils if sleeping is a problem.

Relaxing bath oils for evening use:

Lavender	*3 drops*
Marjoram	*2 drops*
Sandalwood	*1 drop*
Chamomile	*1 drop*
Lavender	*3 drops*
Ylang ylang	*2 drops*

Relaxing bath oils for morning use:

Lavender	*3 drops*
Bergamot	*2 drops*
Geranium	*3 drops*
Juniper	*1 drop*
Lavender	*1 drop*

For people who have difficulty in sleeping, an aromatic bath could be followed by using a few drops of a relaxing essential oil with more sedative properties such as chamomile, lavender, marjoram, ylang ylang or sandalwood inside the pillow slip.

3. Massage with Relaxing Oils

One way of helping someone to relax using aromatherapy is to make up a massage oil using the person's favourite relaxing essential oils. A combination of two or three relaxing essential oils are usually better than a single oil. Massage does not have to be a full body massage to be relaxing. A fifteen minute hand or foot massage or head and scalp massage can have amazing effects.

Here are some of the ways in which massage has been used to promote relaxation:

Theory into Practice

1. To Promote Sleep

Michael is a 28 year old man who has learning difficulties and attends the local training centre. Michael is extremely active and appears to find it very difficult to concentrate on one thing for any length of time or to relax. He is described as having 'autistic tendencies' and he spends most of his time on his own, not communicating with other people.

Michael has had aromatherapy sessions for the past three years and is massaged on a treatment couch at the centre. Staff feel that these sessions have been of considerable benefit to him. Clary sage was found to be the oil which really helped Michael to relax. By vaporising the oil as well as using it in a massage oil he became quiet and relaxed. Staff also noticed that he remained calm and could concentrate more easily in subsequent sessions during the day. Essential oils were introduced at home and Michael's mother stated that she noticed a remarkable difference in his behaviour. He was not as restless and actually slept through the night, whereas before he had had many restless nights. One night Michael's mother heard him enter her room and he stood at the end of her bed holding his bottle of clary sage. She followed him back to his room and massaged his back with the massage oil and Michael was asleep within fifteen minutes.

2. To Reduce Anxiety

Gloria is a 55 year old woman who lives in a hostel. She uses a wheelchair, cannot communicate verbally and is completely dependent on other people for her personal needs. Gloria appears to be very anxious - she continually puts her hands to her ears, grinds her teeth and moves her head from side to side in an agitated manner. She occasionally goes to the pub but has few other occasions when she goes into the community.

At her Individual Planning meeting it was decided to look at different ways to help her to relax using local community resources. A local aromatherapist was found whose home was wheelchair accessible and an appointment made. When Gloria arrived for her first session she seemed to be very anxious, grinding her teeth and covering her ears with her hands. With the key worker a personal history was given including significant illnesses and operations, general health, sleeping patterns, diet and lifestyle information. Gloria has a very dry skin, so a carrier oil containing 10% wheatgerm oil was used.

As the main aim of her session was to help her to relax, Gloria was offered three different relaxing essential oils to smell. She was offered a floral fragrance - lavender, a woody fragrance - sandalwood and a citrus fragrance - bergamot. Gloria has no verbal communication but appeared to prefer the smell of lavender. She turned her head away at the fragrance of sandalwood, made no movements when smelling bergamot but moved closer to smell lavender. The aromatherapist massaged Gloria's feet, legs, back, hands and arms but as Gloria did not appear to enjoy having her face touched, her face and neck were not massaged.

During the session Gloria did not grind her teeth at all and after ten minutes relaxed her hands by her sides. By the time her key worker came to collect her an hour later Gloria was relaxed and asleep. Gloria now receives regular massage and uses lavender in her bath and to scent her room. On subsequent occasions she was given the opportunity to smell other relaxing oils including clary sage, marjoram and ylang ylang. However lavender still appears to be her favourite.

Clive is a 27 year old man who is deaf-blind and who has severe learning and communication difficulties. He is extremely hyperactive and rarely sits still, constantly checking and re-checking his surrounding environment. Although at times, and on his terms, he will accept and/or respond to a hug, he is generally ill-at-ease and distrustful of physical contact.

As a means of relaxing him and gaining his trust, massage was introduced in the form of a daily foot massage which has now progressed to a weekly full body massage. Since starting massage a few months ago, Clive will now usually lie on the massage couch and accept the physical contact for up to thirty minutes. Recently he has started to tolerate having his limbs passively moved to enable the massage therapist to work on the tension held in his upper back, neck and shoulders. The use of essential oils in the massage carrier oil and burner has very much enhanced this work and Clive responds well to their relaxing properties.

3. To Help Reduce Challenging Behaviour

Evelyn is an attractive young lady who is described as being autistic. She attended the 'special care unit' of an adult training centre where she was usually withdrawn, preferring to sit rocking by herself in a corner. When distressed she would bite her hands very badly. She has grand-mal epilepsy and would have a fit on average once every eleven weeks, after which she was often very tense and sore in her shoulders.

Evelyn loves feet and shoes and will often remove people's shoes, collect them in a pile and sit grinning from ear to ear rocking triumphantly. Her key worker decided to introduce massage to improve their relationship, encourage Evelyn to be more involved and to relax and soothe her when she was upset. Her key worker started massaging her feet which she enjoyed and then moved on to her hands, arms, neck and shoulders. Evelyn responded very well, loving the different smells and eventually handed the key worker the bottles of oil and lotions. They built up a close and trusting relationship which affected other activities that they shared. She often initiated a massage session by fetching the oils or offering the key worker her feet. But when the key worker tried to encourage her to massage *her* feet in return, Evelyn ran off delightedly with the key worker's shoes! Interestingly her epilepsy has also improved and Evelyn has even less frequent fits. She has now moved to a new supported home living with a group of autistic adults. She has settled in well and continues to receive and enjoy massage.

Jean. An aromatherapist was invited to spend some time working in a hospital for people with learning difficulties. She began working with a young girl called Jean who appeared to be very disturbed. Jean was continually thrashing backwards and forwards, punching her head with her fists, slapping her head and face, putting her fingers in her eyes and pushing away any hands which tried to touch her. Staff told the aromatherapist that Jean refused to allow people to touch her.

The aromatherapist spent two hours with her using a massage oil made up with relaxing essential oils. At first any contact with Jean was met with total rejection and then, ever so slowly, a gradual acceptance of the aromatherapist's presence took place, leading eventually to the acceptance of touch. During the last half hour of the two hour session Jean appeared relaxed and was lying back in the bean bag, with her arms behind her head smiling and sometimes laughing.

4. To Help Reduce Self Injury

Christopher is a young man with dual sensory impairment. After every meal he would continually regurgitate his food for up to one hour. At one stage he became dangerously ill as a result and had to spend some time in hospital. After this, the support staff where he lived worked out a programme with him to monitor and help reduce this behaviour.

When the massage therapist was invited in, Christopher was still regurgitating although not as severely as before. The massage therapist worked with him weekly, immediately after lunch, to see if massage would make any difference. On the first occasion, Christopher was very wary and kept moving away to regurgitate. The massage therapist noticed that if Christopher was under pressure to conform he regurgitated more. She therefore let him guide the sessions. When he pulled his hands away from her she didn't pull them back, but kept her hands close to his, occasionally gently nudging them or putting them up to his nose so he could smell the oils and to remind him that she was there. Often Christopher would offer his hands again and allow some touch and massage for a short time before pulling away again. Eventually, after about thirty minutes, he moved away completely and refused to join in, so the massage therapist finished the session. In this way she hoped that Christopher would learn that massage was something about which he had a choice.

At the next session, the massage therapist expected to go through the same procedure. However, as soon as Christopher smelled the oils, he laughed, sat down and pulled the massage therapist towards him and offered his hands. He allowed her to massage his hands and then his feet and obviously thoroughly enjoyed the experience, laughing and pulling one hand away and immediately offering the other or stretching a foot out to be massaged. When she lifted his T-shirt to try some back massage, he became quite quiet and still, concentrating on the sensations on his back. The massage therapist noticed that he only regurgitated two or three times in the one hour session.

On another occasion she noticed that when she did relaxing strokes, Christopher settled down and smiled contentedly; when she used more stimulating strokes he became very alert and if she removed her hands he would either replace them or attempt to imitate the stroke himself.

One time the massage therapist combined her work with the programme developed by the support workers in an attempt to cut out the regurgitation completely. Whenever Christopher regurgitated, the support worker would step in and firmly close his mouth, tip his head up, encourage him to swallow and give him a tissue to wipe away the overspill. Interestingly, Christopher regurgitated more in that session than in any of the other massage sessions. The massage work with Christopher continues.

Julie is 26 and lives in the community in her own home supported by residential social workers. Julie has severe learning difficulties, has no verbal communication and is visually impaired. She frequently bites and pinches her arms which are badly scarred as a result. Her support team decided to take Julie to a local aromatherapist to increase her opportunities to be in the community and to help her relax. She attends the aromatherapist on a weekly basis. Initially, the whole session consisted of brief periods of hand massage, as this was all that Julie would tolerate. After a long talk to her keyworker the aromatherapist suggested relaxing oils to be put into Julie's bath, and made up a cream to help reduce scarring.

After six sessions the aromatherapist was able to massage Julie's hands, arms, back and stomach. Julie enjoys this and if the aromatherapist pauses for a moment Julie firmly takes her hands and puts them onto her back or stomach to continue massaging. The aromatherapist has noticed that Julie has started to mimic her movements and will lightly rub or stroke the arm which she usually bites. The support staff have reported that Julie does not bite or scratch her arm as much as she used to and the scars on her arms are noticeably reduced.

5. To Help Release Emotional Tension

A study undertaken using foot massage with people who are in hospital with mental health problems indicated that touching and massage are important in reducing tension. Many similar studies have been carried out by nurses, and Holmes (1986), Sims (1986), and Turton (1989) have all evaluated the therapeutic and relaxing value of massage.

The head, neck, shoulders, back and stomach are common places where tension is stored. Think of the words that are used:

Butterflies in my stomach
I'm all churned up
Get off my back
Carrying the weight of the world on my shoulders
Weighed down by responsibility

Massaging these areas not only relaxes and releases the physical tension that has built up, but may also give the body permission to release the emotional reasons for the physical tension. Tears, therefore, may not be an indication that the person dislikes what you are doing, but may be a necessary part of 'letting go'.

It is important to be sensitive - it is usually clear whether an emotional reaction is a release or an expression of dislike.

Jack is a 21 year old man who is deaf and has severe learning difficulties. He is highly emotional and during emotional outbursts will injure himself. As his only form of communication is a basic knowledge of signing, it is very hard for him to express his sadness or anger to the staff of the home where he lives, or for them to understand him fully .

On many occasions it has been possible to distract Jack from injuring himself by massaging his feet. He now receives a weekly full body massage which is therapeutic for the tension in his shoulders and also gives him a space where he has learned to feel more at ease and able to let go and often cry. Here he can experience the non-sexual yet intimate contact that he would receive from his family if he still had contact with them. He has learned that the massage room is a space that he can use as he wants. If he wants an undisturbed sleep afterwards or a quiet settling time, that will be respected for as long as he needs. After a massage, Jack is noticeably more relaxed and, if not happier, more in contact and aware of himself.

■ In conclusion

Peoples' experiences demonstrate that aromatherapy and massage can help a person to relax. This relaxation works on many levels, not just the physical, and can create a sense of comfort, acceptance and reassurance that can affect the way that the person chooses to respond to different situations in her life.

9

Aromatherapy and Massage to Uplift and Invigorate

Claims that some essential oils uplift and invigorate tired bodies and minds have been made for many centuries.

According to the popular press most members of the royal family use invigorating essential oils to inhale for a quick pick me up. Rosemary is well known for its properties as a mental stimulant and lemon is particularly useful to enliven a tired body.

A Japanese study, recently reported in 'The New Scientist' (August 1990) and conducted in 1988 by Professor Shizuo Torii from Toho University School of Medicine, distinguished between invigorating, stimulating oils and those oils with a calming and sedative action. The researchers tested nineteen different essential oils using a technique which monitored brain patterns. They found that when the subject was presented with the fragrance of an invigorating oil the amplitude of the brain pattern increased. This generally increases when a person is alert and concentrating on something. The stimulant caffeine also increased the reaction time. During the experiment, heart rate and level of sleepiness did not change.

The amplitude of the brain pattern consistently went down when the person was smelling a sedative oil such as lavender. Computer and word processor operators in Japan were found to make 20% fewer errors when exposed to the fragrance of lavender and 54% fewer errors with lemon fragrance.

One of the largest construction companies in Japan is taking these results very seriously and they are now designing offices and hospitals with an 'aroma generation system' to allow fragrances to be piped into the workplace. As a number of oils are known to stimulate the nervous system, it seems reasonable to accept that they would sharpen the mind, thus improving both concentration and memory.

A journalist was given a bottle of rosemary oil to use on a handkerchief whilst typing into the early hours. She later wrote a letter of appreciation to the supplier as it had vastly improved her concentration, enabling her to finish her work much more quickly than usual (Price, S. 1987 Aromanews). It follows that if essential oils can improve and help concentration then a person's memory and learning capacity could be increased.

Research is continuing at many centres in the world, including Warwick University, to look at the possibility of odours being used to improve the memory, as the brain's centre for memory and olfaction are both contained within the same area, the limbic system.

Uplifting oils which can be used where a person suffers from depression include:

Bergamot	*Geranium*
Clary sage	*Lavender*

The most invigorating essential oils which are well known for their clear piercing aromas include:

Eucalyptus	*Peppermint*
Lemon	*Rosemary*

■ Using Uplifting and Invigorating Essential Oils with People who have Learning Difficulties

1. Vaporising Invigorating Oils

Uplifting and invigorating oils can be used to stimulate both mentally and physically. Rosemary and lemon, both mental stimulants, could be vaporised where concentration is required; in the classroom, office, workplace or day centre. When people are required to be physically active, any of the uplifting and invigorating fragrances described can help to create an energetic atmosphere which would be welcomed during a keep fit or physiotherapy session.

Theory into Practice

An occupational therapist regularly held keep fit classes in a local resource centre attended by people who have learning difficulties. She added ten drops of invigorating essential oils to a saucer filled with water and placed it on top of a radiator to create an energetic atmosphere.

2. Using Uplifting and Invigorating Oils in the Bath

Some people find it difficult to get going in the morning and a bath using invigorating oils can help. The effects are usually immediate, and are fully felt up to two hours later. Any of the uplifting or invigorating oils could be used according to the person's personal favourite. The following oil mixes can also be vaporised or used in 2-3 teaspoons of carrier oil or lotion for a massage or application.

Uplifting early morning bath oils:

Bergamot *2 drops*
Rosemary *2 drops*

Invigorating early morning bath oils:

Lemon *1 drop*
Peppermint *1 drop*
Rosemary *3 drops*

Juniper *1 drop*
Lavender *1 drop*
Peppermint *1 drop*
Rosemary *1 drop*

Eucalyptus *1 drop*
Lemon *2 drops*
Geranium *2 drops*

Refreshing bath oils to relieve overworked muscles:

Eucalyptus *1 drop*
Juniper *1 drop*
Lavender *1 drop*
Rosemary *2 drops*

3. Massage with Uplifting and Invigorating Oils

Massage does not always have to be soothing and relaxing. By using quick, brisk strokes and patting or tapping strokes (not normally used in aromatherapy massage) a massage can become an energising experience, particularly when invigorating oils are used to make up the massage oil. Massage with refreshing or invigorating oils can be used to reduce sluggishness either first thing in the morning or at other times of the day. It can also be used to improve responsiveness or involvement in an activity.

Theory into Practice

Catherine is a small fragile woman with multiple disabilities. She spends all her day slumped in a wheelchair at the day centre, apparently lifeless and with little recognisable response to anything. She makes no eye contact. However, when her key worker started massaging her hands Catherine made little moaning noises. If Catherine moved her hands even a little, the key worker responded with her hands and commented on the movements immediately. The key worker gently talked to her all the time and tried to make eye contact, praising her if she did look at her, however fleetingly. She felt that there was definitely some response and felt very heartened when she received an excited letter from Catherine's mother who said, "after 35 years I have never known Catherine to make eye contact. Perhaps there is more there. Perhaps she has been fooling us all this time."

The key worker continued the massage regularly, working on her shoulders and back and encouraged Catherine to sit up. By gradually improving the tone in Catherine's neck muscles she was able to keep her head up for short periods.

10

Interactive Massage

Massage and aromatherapy can help people to learn to trust, share, and interact with each other. The work of J. McGee (1985) and McInnes and Treffry (1982) places the emphasis on developing a valued relationship with the person who has learning difficulties, and seeing this as the primary goal and focus of support and intervention.

Massage is a form of non-verbal communication. It enables the development of positive interactions in a non-verbal and non-threatening way, assisting individuals to become more aware of other people as well as themselves. Massage is known for having 'emotionally releasing effects'. People who generally find it difficult to 'open up' sometimes find that they are able to do so during, or as a result of, massage. For people who have more severe learning difficulties, communication and interaction can be developed through 'Interactive Massage' where the primary focus of massage is to encourage responsiveness, interaction and participation rather than aiming purely at sensory awareness (Multisensory Massage, see Chapter 11), relaxation or invigoration.

■ Massage and Communication

Massage involves a degree of trust and intimacy and can help people develop relationships with each other. It can help a person feel accepted and nurtured. A nurse, working in a general hospital describes how, through massage, a patient felt safe enough to trust her and share her inner feelings (Smith, M. 1990). Many nurses are now beginning to use aromatherapy and massage within hospitals with many benefits. They are becoming aware that massage can help to establish a good rapport with patients, some of whom are able to express themselves in a way they had not felt able to before.

One nurse who works with elderly people said that, "Massage brought many benefits to our patients. Touching in this beautiful and non-sexual way opened the doors to a closer relationship with us, allowing patients to speak of their dreams and hopes, and their fears and pleasures'' (Passant, H. 1990).

A physiotherapist working with people who have anorexia stated that, ''The non-verbal skills of massage, relaxation and movement enable patients to explore inner feelings of self, which they can then talk about'' (Davison, K. 1990).

Theory into Practice

Massage and aromatherapy were used with a woman who has learning difficulties who had recently undergone a hysterectomy. Barbara was obviously distressed by this but appeared to find it difficult to talk about. She was also worried about her mother who had a serious illness. Barbara attended a local adult training centre and to help her relax her key worker began massaging her hands and feet on a daily basis in a small quiet room at the Centre. In the calm environment, and whilst receiving a relaxing massage, Barbara began to open up about her fears for the future regarding her mother's illness in a way in which the keyworker believed would not have occurred in a counselling session.

An occupational therapist describes how she used massage and aromatherapy to 'get to know' people who have severe learning difficulties and who cannot communicate verbally. When a person is referred to her she spends the first few sessions just massaging their hands before beginning other forms of support and intervention.

Paul lives in a hospital with other people who have learning difficulties. He has frequent epileptic fits and spends most of the day on the ward shouting and grinding his teeth. He appears to have very little interest in doing any activity. Although in general Paul dislikes being touched he is very tolerant of massage. During a massage he will look at the person who is massaging him, whereas usually, he rarely looks at people or makes contact with their eyes. There is a noticeable difference in his behaviour after the occupational therapist has massaged his face, neck and feet. He no longer grinds his teeth or shouts but appears calmer and his breathing is more regular.

Hand massage is sometimes used in team building and experiential group work to encourage trust and sharing together. In a similar way it can be used in drama sessions or other workshops to enable people to experience the giving and receiving of a hand massage and turn taking.

We have already discussed the importance of supporting and enabling people with learning difficulties to communicate and develop relationships. As these examples show, massage can help to improve eye contact, strengthen and develop relationships and help people to 'open up'.

■ Gentle Teaching

Gentle Teaching places an emphasis on the development of relationships. It was created by Dr. John McGee, a psychologist from Nebraska and his colleagues. His work is based on humanistic philosophy, believing that people have an inherent value which is not based on achievement or possessions. Some people with learning difficulties may exhibit challenging behaviour, behaving in a way that injures themselves or is destructive or anti-social. McGee suggests that such behaviour is not challenging or difficult but distressed and angry.

Gentle Teaching is a teaching process which places bonding and the development of relationships at the centre of human development. It is based upon the premise that within each individual there is a longing for union with others. Many people who have learning difficulties may not be aware of this longing as it may exist at a subconscious level.

There are only a few 'techniques' of Gentle Teaching. Touch is used as a method of demonstrating a belief in the person's value, and to develop a warm relationship. McGee describes the use of 'tactile strokes' in the case of Sam who was diagnosed as being severely 'retarded' and autistic, with self-injurious behaviour. During his Gentle Teaching sessions his caregiver blocked attempts at self-injury and provided one-to-one support, redirecting Sam to participate in tasks. Sam was given praise and affectionate 'tactile strokes' for small amounts of involvement in the task (Brandon, D. 1990).

Gentle Teaching stresses the need to move away from relationships in which the support worker has the authority and power, and to focus on developing value and relationships with people who have learning difficulties, from which real learning can occur.

■ The Interactive Sequence and Interactive Massage

McInnes and Treffry (1982) offer a similar approach, which stresses the importance of a relationship, stating that the objective of all activities should be promoting the growth of a bond between the intervenor and child. They illustrate this with an eight stage sequence which we have termed the 'Interactive Sequence'. Their work is the result of years of involvement with children who have visual and auditory impairment or, to use their words, who are 'multisensorily deprived'. They suggest that it is only through a close relationship that a multisensorily deprived (the preferred term is now dual sensory impairment) child will be motivated to explore the environment.

> You will provide the motivation which will encourage the child to reach outside himself and to initiate interaction between himself and the environment.[1]

Bronfenbrenner (1974) also suggests that the primary objective of intervention should be the establishment of an enduring emotional relationship.

McInnes and Treffry suggest that this relationship will be most likely to be established by physical contact, encouraging the person to tolerate and later enjoy this interaction more than any self stimulating or challenging behaviours which the person may have developed. It may take weeks or even months before the person begins to relax and enjoy the contact, but this will be the basis for future growth and development. It is anticipated that there are eight stages that the person may progress through before this will happen.

1 Resists
2 Tolerates
3 Co-operates passively
4 Enjoys
5 Responds co-operatively
6 Leads
7 Imitates
8 Initiates

1. McInnes, J. Treffry, J. 1982

Interactive Massage involves supporting a person with severe learning difficulties to work through this sequence. Initially when massage is introduced to a person, she may be resistant and hide her hands. Proponents of Gentle Teaching suggest that a high degree of tolerance and warmth is required on the part of the carer, who may receive kicks, scratches and screams when an activity is introduced. McInnes and Treffry suggest that you do not insist but switch to a related activity you know she enjoys.

From this stage of resistance, the person will be able to tolerate the massage for short periods, fleetingly initially, progressing to a number of minutes, until she co-operates passively with the massage and later begins to show signs of enjoyment. In the fifth stage, which is 'responds co-operatively', the person will cease to be just a passive recipient but will begin to respond co-operatively offering her hands and selecting creams and oils. From this stage she may begin to lead the session, anticipating the sequence and direction of the activity. The next stage involves the person beginning to imitate the carer's movements either on the back of her own hands or beginning to rub the carer's hands. At the final stage she will initiate the session independently, finding the massage oil or indicating that she wants a massage.

Gentle Teaching stresses the importance of equality in relationships but, as this sequence shows, at the start of the relationship with people with learning difficulties, giving and receiving are often imbalanced. The support worker or carer initially gives much more and appears to receive little. As the relationship develops this is redressed as the individual becomes more responsive and involved in the relationship, which is the goal of Interactive Massage.

Theory into Practice

Warren is a young man who is very hyperactive and finds it difficult to settle. Staff at the day centre couldn't get him involved in any group work and his concentration was limited to things he really enjoyed on a one-to-one basis such as playing rough and tumble, or ball games or going to the disco. Massage was introduced to try to develop a stronger relationship with Warren and to encourage him to concentrate on another activity. His key worker took him to a quiet room where there were mats and started massaging his hands, but after a few seconds he would pull away and run off (Stage 1 - Resists). She never pulled him back but made the sessions very frequent even if short. Gradually he began to like the smell of the relaxing essential oils, and tolerated touch for longer sessions (Stage 2 - Tolerates).

He began to enjoy the sessions (Stage 3 - Enjoys) and became quite adept at showing what he wanted, proffering an arm or rolling onto his front and baring his back (Stage 5 - Responds Co-operatively). Warren eventually enjoyed sessions of up to 45 minutes of massage and developed a good and trusting relationship with his key worker which was maintained in other things that they did together. He would often lead a session (Stage 6 - Leads) and even initiate it by fetching the oils from a drawer or leading the key worker into the quiet room (Stage 8 - Initiates). At the end of the sessions he was more relaxed. One day the key worker was massaging the hands of another student and Warren wanted to join in. She gave him some hand lotion and he rubbed it carefully into the other student's hands (Stage 7 - Imitates).

An occupational therapist and trainee psychologist set up a basic stimulation and awareness workshop to assess the needs of a group of people living in a hospital for whom there was no appropriate day care. These people were considered either too physically disabled or challenging to fit into existing day service provision and so spent all day, every day, on the ward. A multi-sensory programme was introduced to help the therapists gain an understanding of each individual and assess each one's likes and dislikes. They found that relaxing and invigorating massage used within the framework of McInnes and Treffry's interactive sequence was a valuable and therapeutic tool to help them develop a relationship with each person and interpret any communication. The sessions were assessed weekly and evaluated every three months. The following examples describe how two people responded and benefited from the approach.

Samantha has lived in institutions since birth and has a low level of tolerance to touch. She has no verbal communication and spends all day on the ward in a wheelchair which she propels with her foot or hand. She is a determined woman with a strong personality and clear ideas about what she wants. She spends a lot of time playing with objects that click or rattle. Essential oils of peppermint (to aid her digestion), basil (for invigoration) and lemon (to reduce the oedema in her legs) were used in a carrier oil of wheatgerm, avocado and grapeseed oils. Initially she resisted any contact after only a few seconds. But after three months of patient regular persistence, Samantha began to enjoy having her hands touched and began to initiate the use of some musical instruments - a tambourine and xylophone. At this point a computer was introduced with a single touch switch which, when activated, immediately gave visual feedback. At first, Samantha co-operated passively but after several weeks she started to lead the session, wheeling herself over to the computer. She would also initiate the massage, stretching out to hold the therapist's arm. She now visits a college twice a week where she attends a computer course and is a member of a communication group.

Julie is 47 years old, has no known relatives and has lived in institutions since she was 5 years old. She has severe kyphoscoliosis to the right and no hip movements, no verbal communication, is resistant to using her hands and spends all day in a semi-reclined position. She is unable to eat independently and generally lacks sensory stimulation. She enjoys listening to classical music.

Invigorating oils of peppermint, basil and lemon were vaporised and used in a massage oil to stimulate Julie and to improve her circulation and digestion. The main purposes of each session were to encourage Julie to use her hands to develop communication and to increase her tolerance of touch. She was placed over a wedge to encourage a more functional position. Julie was initially totally resistant during the first session but gradually allowed her hands to be massaged for increasing periods; from just two minutes on the back of her hands she came to enjoy a full hand massage on each hand lasting fifteen to twenty minutes.

The therapist's understanding of her non-verbal communication increased greatly. As her touch tolerance increased, Julie learned how to switch on her classical music tape by reaching out and operating a single box switch. She began to initiate hand massage by reaching out and would also massage the therapist's hands and maintain eye contact. All these developments are continuing to be used to widen Julie's experience and to help her to do more for herself.

Walter is 42 years old, with elective mutism and a low tolerance of touch. He is very tense and anxious and this is reflected in his posture; he sits with fists clenched, arms folded and legs tightly crossed, grinding his teeth. Consequently activities like eating independently and drinking are very difficult. He has lived in institutions since he was 18 years old. His parents visited him weekly and took him out for a drink which he enjoyed. However, they both recently died and Walter has been understandably upset and disorientated. Massage was introduced, and relaxing oils of chamomile, geranium and lavender were used to help deal with his presenting problems.

Walter spent a day each week at a semi-detached house used for training by the Occupational Therapy Department and massage was started there. Initially Walter would only tolerate his arms and shoulders being rubbed for three minutes. By six weeks he was co-operating passively, allowing foot and hand massage, but sitting up so that his body was not fully relaxed. Six months later he would lie down fully and respond co-operatively to massage. His whole body would begin to relax and he would keep his arms unfolded throughout the 30 minute session. It has also had a good effect on his eating. Whereas before Walter ate at a special table with protection on the floor, a cushion behind his back, a built up spoon, sunflower plate and dycem mat; now he sits at an ordinary table, uses an ordinary spoon and only needs a plate guard. He no longer needs a cushion or the floor covering. He has just started attending a college of tertiary education one day per week.

A teacher describes how an Interactive Massage programme was used to develop emotional bonding with a child who has severe learning difficulties and sensory disabilities. She suggests that without emotional bonding a child will not attempt to communicate and that massage gave this child that 'certain something' for which it was worth communicating. Initially this communication was just a smile when stroked (Stage 4 - Enjoys) but later this developed to the point where the child found the bottle of massage oil, went to the adult and took her to the area where the massage session usually took place (Stage 8 -Initiates).

Another child who was in the Resist Stage (Stage 1) took well over six months to relax sufficiently to allow the teacher to massage her.

This later led to the child taking a more active role, moving from resisting (Stage 1) to tolerating (Stage 2), co-operating passively (Stage 3) and then responding co-operatively (Stage 5). Over the next two years of Interactive Massage sessions the teacher describes how the child began to develop an awareness of her own body and joined in 'body games' such as 'your hand, my hand' (Stage 7 - Imitates).

Interactive Massage places the emphasis on encouraging the person and giving her opportunities to respond, lead, imitate and initiate massage, rather than using massage solely to relax the person and expecting her to receive it passively. The Interactive Sequence presents us with progressive, recognisable stages. These can be used to assess the progress made by people with severe and profound learning difficulties as they learn to interact with others and develop relationships.

The Interactive Sequence

	Stage	Description of Response	Example: Hand Massage
Passive Massage	**1.** Resists	Initially resists the activity. Do not insist, but switch to a related activity which you know the person enjoys. Return to the new activity once the tension has disappeared.	Person initially tries to resist and hides her hands. Switch to touch which you know she enjoys, eg. stroke hair, arms. Try again.
	2. Tolerates	Is able to tolerate activity for a period of time because of the rewarding one-to-one contact rather than the activity itself. Gradually tolerates activity for longer periods.	Will allow support worker to touch her hands fleetingly. This is extended until the support worker can touch and stroke her hands for five minutes without the person withdrawing her hands.
	3. Co-operates passively	Support worker will notice a subtle change in response as the person becomes less resistant.	Person allows her hands to be massaged for longer periods; different strokes can be introduced.
	4. Enjoys	Person becomes more relaxed and familiar with the activity. Remains passive but demonstrates signs of enjoyment.	Person may smile when she is touched or stroked.
Interactive Massage	**5.** Responds co-operatively	Person will follow the support worker's lead with little direction or need for encouragement.	Person will begin to smile and show signs of enjoyment when the bottle of cream or oil is given to her, and will proffer her hands for the massage to begin.
	6. Leads	Person will begin to anticipate the sequence and direction of the activity.	Person will show that she is aware that you have finished massaging one hand and will offer the other.
	7. Imitates	Person will go through the sequence of activity independently, given appropriate communication.	Person may begin to imitate the support worker's strokes on the back of her own hands.
	8. Imitates independently	Person will imitate activity without prompting.	Person takes bottle of oil to the support worker at the time when the massage usually begins. Reciprocal massage can be introduced where person rubs cream into support worker's hands after massage.

11

Multisensory Massage

Multisensory Massage is the use of different textures, tools, talcs, lotions and oils fragranced with essential oils to provide stimulation to the senses. Individuals who have severe and profound learning difficulties are constantly touched in a variety of ways. One person's hands may be responsible for dressing and removing clothing, another pair of hands may clean and wash, and yet other hands move the person from bed to chair or toilet. Massage is a valuable way in which relaxing, calming and soothing touch can be experienced.

As well as an increased understanding of human touch, experience needs to be gained of other tactile activities in a learning environment using a sensory development approach. Often physical limitations, a lack of motivation or opportunity can prevent the person from reaching out, touching, exploring, gathering and interpreting information from the environment. Without this, she will be unable to respond to the environment or learn that she can have an effect on it. People may need support in experiencing different textures and tactile objects, as well as understanding human touch. This can be encouraged through the use of Multisensory Massage.

Multisensory Massage can be used in schools within the science programme of the National Curriculum, in Attainments 1a1 and 1a3, which involve reacting to sensory stimulation and showing interest in, and exploring materials.

■ Developing Tactile Experiences through Multisensory Massage

Flo Longhorn (1988) suggests several aims which could be incorporated into a Tactile Curriculum to help children become more aware of their environment.

These aims include:

a Increasing awareness of tactile experiences. Simple discrimination skills form the beginnings of an awareness of the characteristics of different objects.

b An increased tolerance of touch, which can help individuals feel more at ease with positioning and handling. Events such as having toe nails cut may become less distressing.

Hand and arm massage can help to facilitate manual manipulation as a prelude to formal signing and finger spelling. Massage can help children who are resistant to having their hands touched and shaped into signs.

c An improved awareness of an individual's own body. For some people this may involve the beginnings of a positive body image. Individuals who have learning difficulties may have had very little nourishing contact when young, leading to a poor body image. Massage is a recognised way of helping someone to become aware that their body is valuable and worth taking care of.

Working with people who have anorexia, a physiotherapist described how using massage with oils can give a sense of well-being and self-worth, to show that the patient's body is worth massaging even if the person herself may hate her own body (Davison, K. 1990).

Longhorn (1988) suggests that an awareness of different parts of her body may help a child avoid a painful experience. For example she may be aware of the need to move her leg away from a hot radiator. Such an objective-based approach is useful. Yet it is a meaningless and impossible task to analyse every area of responsiveness to touch. Fun, enjoyment and the provision of a wide range of opportunity to experience and explore touch provide a firm foundation for other learning experiences.

■ Using Multisensory Massage

To develop this positive awareness of touch, textures and smells, Multisensory Massage can be used in conjunction with other activities which provide opportunities for sensory experiences.

■ Using Textures and Tools within Multisensory Massage

There are many commercial tools available for massage which can be purchased at large chemists or health shops, including the following:

Body Buddy	*a textured rubber mitt*
Massage band	*made from rough texture hemp*
Mini Masseur	*a wooden massage roller*
Electric massagers	*there are several electric massagers available with interchangeable heads which incorporate many textures*

Different textures can also be used, for example:

Velvet	*Cotton wool*
Sponge	*Wool*
Soft brushes	*Silky material*
Natural bristle brushes	*Flannel*

A portable foot spa is a useful way of incorporating vibration and water and is also wonderfully relaxing. Incorporating textures or tools into a massage can be done before, after or instead of a massage with oils or lotion. For example, a multisensory foot massage may begin by gently rubbing the feet with a piece of velvet, after which a soft brush could be used, followed by rubbing with silky material. This could be followed by ten minutes in the footspa using relaxing essential oils before gently drying the feet on a soft towel and massaging with oil which contains the same essential oils.

Theory into practice

Sue is a 6 year old girl who attends a school for children with profound learning difficulties. The community occupational therapist visits the school to help Sue to improve her head control, visual attention, choice making, hand function and hand-eye coordination. The teachers use a 'Holistic Sensory Approach' (Sanderson, H., Gitsham, N. 1990) which, by concentrating on using the senses expands Sue's awareness of herself and the environment. The physiotherapist runs a 'Hand Class' which concentrates on grasping and releasing objects, and Sue's teacher plays hand games and sings action songs with her.

Multisensory Massage sessions are used by the occupational therapist (O.T.) to help Sue use her hands to explore her environment. The O.T. begins the multisensory massage session by gently rubbing Sue's hand with a soft bristle shaving brush for a minute. Sue appears to like this and giggles. This is followed by using a flannel massage mit which has a foam covering on one side and cotton flannel on the other. After the contrasting textures of the foam, flannel and brush, soft velvet is used. Sue seems to prefer softer textures to others. The session is completed by gently massaging both of Sue's hands with talc for ten minutes and finishing with a hand massage using invigorating essential oils. This session occurs two mornings a week directly before lunch, to loosen Sue's hands. This helps her to use her padded spoon more easily.

Steven is a 23 year old man who has lived in a large institution since he was 5 years old. He was diagnosed at 5 months old as having encephalitis which has resulted in him having epilepsy, cortical blindness and severe learning difficulties. Twelve months ago he moved out of the institution into a small group home. He now attends a small day unit for people who have a visual impairment. An RNIB assessment reported that Steven had potentially useful vision and responded to light.

The O.T. used the 'Kidderminster Curriculum for Children and Adults with Profound Multiple Learning Difficulties' as it provided a list of events that appeared to be reinforcing for Steven. By using this it was found that he enjoyed music, hugs and vibration. From the beginning of the sessions it was obvious that he enjoyed physical contact, but would resist any attempt to encourage the use of his hands to explore anything in his environment.

Multisensory Massage was used and many different textures were given to Steven to encourage him to explore with his hands. Using an Interactive Massage approach, the O.T. encouraged Steven to use his hands. Gradually instead of remaining passive and occasionally pushing objects away if he didn't like them, Steven would move the O.T.'s hand to the object he wanted. The favourite object was a Pifco body massager. The O.T. used a relaxing oil with essential oils of geranium, lavender and marjoram. After four sessions he began to recognise the noise of the body massager vibrating on the floor and would giggle. If the massager was near him he would reach out and hold it, drawing it towards his body. By using an adapted switch the O.T. aims to help Steven learn how to switch the massager on and off himself. Then, perhaps, he could learn to generalise this in order to enable him to switch things on and off in the home, giving him more choice and control in his environment.

■ Using Multisensory Massage to Decrease Intolerance of Touch

Some individuals have a poor tolerance of touch, which can make positioning and moving uncomfortable. For some people any form of touch can be extremely unpleasant. McInnes and Treffry (1982) describe the behaviour of some children who are multisensorily deprived because of dual sensory impairment. They are:

> ...like erratic butterflies which never light for more than an instant. Often they don't like to be held or touched, avoid giving eye contact and refuse to interact with peers or adults. Some children exhibit reactions to clothing either because of their hyperactive-like activity or because sensory damage has caused a very low threshold of tolerance to tactile sensations.

Ayres (1972) noted similar behaviour in other children and adults who did not have visual or auditory impairment, and suggested that a child who is hyperactive and easily distracted may be 'tactile defensive'.

Knickerbocker (1980) suggests that an individual who is intolerant of touch has heightened sensitivity to information about touch and tactile experiences because there is an imbalance between the inhibitory and excitatory forces within the nervous system. There is too little inhibition and the sensory message is transmitted too easily, so that an excess of sensory information floods the higher centres of the central nervous system. As this sensory information is not properly monitored or suitably integrated with other sensory information, it becomes overwhelming for the individual and causes her to react excessively when touched.

An individual who is intolerant of touch may withdraw by moving quickly away from touch whilst registering an anxious expression. This adverse reaction is normal in toddlers who are tired and therefore irritable, but a child who cannot tolerate touch may react in this way regularly and consistently. Light touch will be found to be excessively ticklish so that sometimes the individual will remove clothing. A person who is intolerant of touch may wear long sleeves only in order to keep her arms covered and therefore less vulnerable. This behaviour can eventually have profound effects on development. It has been found that children may be unable to develop a good body image and spatial awareness. Hand function may be affected together with a tendency to retreat away from interpersonal contact and communication.

McInnes and Treffry (1982) suggest that the child should be exposed to sensory input at a level which she can assimilate and as her tolerance grows the type and strength of stimulation can be increased. Knickerbocker suggests that an individual will progress through the following stages:

1 Rejects human contact
2 Accepts being touched by people she can trust
3 Avoids textures due to a feeling of discomfort on her hands
4 Initiates touching

Multisensory Massage can play a vital role in working to decrease intolerance of touch. Although initially the individual will reject massage, by slowly progressing through the Interactive Sequence, she will come to a stage where she will tolerate being touched by familiar people. Once that stage has been accomplished textures can be incorporated into the massage as described earlier until the individual will initiate touching, and Interactive Massage can take place.

Theory into Practice

Shaun has dual sensory impairment. He pulled away from people so that it was difficult to encourage him to do things for himself. He didn't like having his nails cut and the staff where he lived wanted to introduce a signing programme so he could make his needs known and they could communicate to him on his hands. Massage was introduced to help Shaun work through his intolerance of touch.

He always kept one hand up by his face to protect himself, so the massage therapist worked first on his other hand, gradually building up his trust and taking it at his pace. He slowly started to accept some touch to his protecting hand and would keep it down for short periods. Now he is accepting more touch and is learning basic signs. He smiles when the staff do an 'M' for massage on his hand, signalling the beginning of a massage, and now tolerates having his nails cut.

Louise is a 34 year old woman who lives in a hospital. Not being able to tolerate touch presented Louise with many problems and meant that learning to perform certain skills was more difficult. She has no vision and relies on her sense of touch to identify objects in her environment. Massage with relaxing oils was introduced to increase Louise's tolerance and acceptance of touch.

Louise was initially resistant to being touched but gradually was able to tolerate hand massage for up to five minutes. She also began to handle objects which were given to her. This enabled her to accept being touched and to touch objects more easily.

12

Aromatherapy and Massage to Improve Health

Increasing numbers of people are turning to natural or complementary medicines. In a recent survey conducted by The Journal of Complementary and Alternative Medicine at an alternative medicine exhibition, eight out of ten people said that they would rather use complementary therapies, where possible, than mainstream medicines. This is beginning to be acknowledged by the medical professions with a consultant neurologist recently saying, "Individuals are showing less willingness to trust medical authority, and are searching for ways to (better) health by improved nutrition and fitness, and holistic therapies".

The Surgeon General in the United States has stated that the use of Aromatherapy should not be discouraged, and our own Chief Medical Officer, when talking about people who have AIDS, stated that, "Any psycho-social therapy, particularly involving touch, would be of great benefit".

As well as being able to help the many illnesses which are related to stress through the use of relaxing essential oils it is widely recognised that many other minor conditions can benefit from massage and aromatherapy. These minor disorders include aches and pains, digestive difficulties, pre-menstrual tension, skin conditions and minor infections such as a sore throat or cystitis. Research by dermatologists has shown that a 5% dilution of essential oil of tea tree is as effective in the treatment of acne as Benzoyl Peroxide, yet is kinder to the skin. The researchers describe tea tree oil as being, "a valuable alternative to orthodox treatment" (The Lancet, 1990, Vol. 336, p1438).

More serious conditions and acute illnesses should always be treated medically. Some long term chronic disorders can find a measure of relief through aromatherapy and massage. For example painful joints caused by arthritis could be eased by gentle massage with essential oils.

Essential oils have not been found to react adversely with any chemical drugs and are also compatible with other branches of natural medicine. One exception to this has been suggested in the case of homoeopathy where the strong scent of one or two essential oils (especially eucalyptus and peppermint) may counteract the effects of the remedies, though this is not certain.

■ Using Essential Oils to Improve the Health of People who have Learning Difficulties

Essential oils can be used effectively in many different ways:

1. Improving the Body's General Ability to Combat Infection

Essential oils have been proven to protect the body by stimulating its own natural defences, thus improving resistance to disease. They work by stimulating the immune system through increasing the body's ability to produce white blood cells, which destroy bacteria. Some essential oils stimulate the body's production of white blood cells to a greater degree than others and are known to be immuno-stimulants (Rovesti 1971). The following oils can strengthen the immune system whether they are inhaled or applied to the skin through massage:

Bergamot
Chamomile
Lavender
Lemon
Tea tree

If a person regularly succumbs to infections and colds, using these immunostrengthening oils could help to build the body's natural defences. The oils could be used in the bath on a regular basis or in a massage oil. Massage on its own or enhanced with essential oils stimulates the body's circulation and lymphatic systems to flush toxins and waste from the body. It is helpful if the person can be given a long drink (preferably water) after the massage to help flush those substances away. This will help to prevent headaches and tiredness which may occur from the release of stored toxins into the circulatory system.

Theory into Practice

Staff at an adult training centre noticed that there were always certain students who were more likely to catch colds or infections that were going around the centre. One student with physical disabilities frequently had colds which always went onto her chest. As she didn't have the strength to cough up the phlegm the infections often lasted for weeks. Regular massage to her back, arms and the top of her chest helped to loosen and strengthen the muscles between her ribs so that she could breathe more deeply and cough up more easily. It also helped to loosen the catarrh and improved her lymphatic and circulatory systems which increased her own natural resistance to infections.

2. Promoting the Growth of Healthy New Cells

Lavender has been shown to stimulate the growth of new healthy skin to produce rapid healing. It is used in the burns units of some hospitals for this purpose (Price, S. 1988 Aromanews). Its anti-inflammatory effects also prevent swelling and further infection, properties shared by chamomile and bergamot.

3. Reducing Pain

A very tiny amount of lavender or tea tree applied neat to a bee or wasp sting will bring relief. Although in themselves essential oils are not very strong pain killers they do appear to enhance the body's ability to cope with pain. The most effective oils to help to relieve pain include:

Bergamot
Chamomile
Juniper
Lavender
Marjoram
Rosemary

They have been used in this way for many years - ask any pharmacist for some help with toothache and he or she will probably suggest essential oil of cloves. Compresses made from chamomile can help to treat earache, and sprains or minor wounds can benefit from lavender.

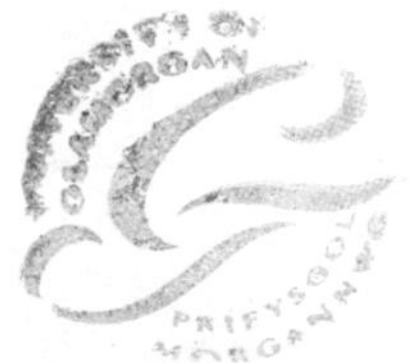

Theory into Practice

Bernita describes herself as middle aged. She has lived in hospitals for most of her life and is now preparing for life in the community. Aromatherapy and its benefits were explained to her and a demonstration of hand massage given. She was initially uncertain but thought that on her hands, which have rheumatism with stiffness and a little pain in them, it would be useful.

The nurse, also an aromatherapist, mixed oils for arthritis and rheumatism to massage Bernita's hands. She regularly treats Bernita's hands, encouraging her to sit comfortably and to relax whilst the hand massage takes place. Bernita relaxes, becomes calm and often smiles during the sessions, saying that her hands appear to be less stiff and more mobile.

The nurse suggested that other parts of the body might be tried and on her fourth visit Bernita was experiencing a migraine with visual disturbance. She accepted a tissue with lavender oil from which to inhale and a gentle massage to the temples, again using lavender but in a carrier oil. Bernita stated that this relieved the pain. However, Bernita continued to want only her hands massaged until three sessions later. On this occasion the nurse used the oils for arthritis and rheumatism on the knees of a staff member. Bernita volunteered that the nurse could do her 'bad knee'. Whilst her knee was being massaged Bernita relaxed almost immediately and remained that way until the nurse left, sometime later.

Bernita now enjoys both her hands and knees being massaged. Perhaps in time Bernita will be happy to accept aromatherapy for other parts of her body, but it has been important to respect her very firm wishes and give her time to adjust to the new experience.

4. Attacking Bacteria, Fungi and Viruses Directly

Another way in which essential oils can improve health is by attacking bacteria and viruses directly, as virtually all essential oils are active against certain infecting organisms. Viruses are thought to cause or be involved in exacerbating the common cold and diseases such as some forms of cancer. Tea tree, lavender and lemon are effective against many different viruses. Most oils are bactericidal and some oils are effective against a wide range of infecting organisms. The following oils all have particular antiseptic and bactericidal properties:

Bergamot	*Lavender*
Eucalyptus	*Rosemary*
Juniper	*Tea tree*

Lavender and tea tree are effective against fungal infections and are therefore useful in treating infections such as athletes foot, using a footbath. Using essential oils in the bath is an excellent way of treating infections such as cystitis. If someone suffers from nasal congestion, decongestant oils such as eucalyptus or peppermint could help. Putting a few drops of either of these oils on a handkerchief inside the pillow slip or in a burner at night could help the person to sleep.

Theory into Practice

Peter is a young man with learning difficulties who lives in a hospital. He suffers from severe nasal congestion and refuses to be touched by anyone apart from two staff whom he knows well. Staff had been using the usual medicines which are used to clear congestion without any success and Peter was keeping others as well as himself awake at night with his breathing difficulties. Recently he had been taken to a specialist in another hospital but as Peter would not let the consultant examine him properly, he had to be brought back without being helped.

The aromatherapist used essential oils for sinus problems on a tissue which was held near his face. At the same time she massaged his feet with the same essential oils in a massage oil, concentrating on the parts of the feet which corresponded to the sinuses. Before beginning this she talked to Peter gently and began by lightly touching and stroking his hands and feet. To the staff's amazement after a while Peter's sinuses began to run.

During a summer playscheme a group of helpers regularly looked after a three year old child with asthma who has a tendency to chesty coughs and infections. One afternoon he was very wheezy and refused his lunch. One of the helpers gave him a massage with bergamot and sprayed the room with a solution of water and bergamot. He lay, playing on the mat and then vomited a small amount of clear fluid twice. After crying for a few minutes he slept for twenty minutes. On waking he finished his lunch enthusiastically and appeared to enjoy a music session. More importantly there was no wheeze or chesty sound. On previous occasions he had always required a nebuliser.

James has learning difficulties and attends his local day centre. Although he is unable to speak, James makes his needs known by using Makaton sign language. When anxious and distressed he makes repetitive noises. The main aim of aromatherapy with James was to treat his skin problem, as he had severe acne and blemishes on his face and back. The day centre officer used essential oil of lavender in a carrier oil to help his skin. It took a few months of regular massage before much success was seen. One year later James' skin remains clear. The lavender massage oil was also used at home and it was noted that James' repetitive noises, indicating he was anxious, had significantly decreased.

5. Preventing the Spread of Infection

Because essential oils are both volatile and antiseptic they are ideal weapons against air borne infection. In the John Radcliffe Hospital in Oxford, oils of geranium, lavender and tea tree are being used instead of chemical disinfectants and antiseptics. All essential oils are antiseptic to some degree with the most potent being:

Bergamot *Lemon*
Eucalyptus *Rosemary*
Juniper *Sandalwood*
Lavender *Tea tree*

Where there is a high risk of infection or an epidemic, the spread of infection can be decreased by vaporising oils such as bergamot, eucalyptus or lavender.

Theory into Practice

On a holiday with six children who have severe learning difficulties, all of whom were prone to chest infections, the nurse sprayed every room each afternoon with a solution of eucalyptus and peppermint. The one day on which the rooms were not sprayed three children and two staff indicated the beginnings of a cold or sore throat. These symptoms disappeared after the rooms were sprayed again.

■ Using Massage to Improve the Health of People Who Have Learning Difficulties.

1. To Improve Circulation

The body has a very good pump, the heart, to make sure that via the circulation of blood, each part of the body receives the nutrients and oxygen it needs to function efficiently. However, through lack of exercise, poor diet, stress and poor posture this system can fail to work as efficiently as it should. In particular the return of blood from different parts of the body back to the heart and lungs can become sluggish. Consequently people may develop circulatory problems such as cold hands and feet, arthritis, varicose veins etc. By always massaging upwards, towards the heart (e.g. from the feet firmly up the legs; from the hands up the arms; from the lower back up to the neck) with firm strokes, some of these conditions can be improved. Feet and hands become warmer and people with arthritis can experience relief from pain and stiffness, because improved circulation to the joints reduces inflammation and pain.

Theory into Practice

Philippa is a young woman who has Downs Syndrome. She has dry skin and stiff and painful joints. Her knees are particularly swollen, red and painful, so the massage therapist worked on her legs above the sensitive area, improving the circulation in them, relaxing the muscles and improving the lymph drainage. Within twenty minutes of massage two or three times a week Philippa felt a great improvement. The staff at the day centre noticed that she was walking more easily and with less pain. The massage therapist also used massage and shiatsu points on her hands and arms to relieve stiffness and improve circulation. Starting to use Interactive Massage she asked Philippa one day if she would like to try massaging the therapist's hands. Philippa did so, carefully and sensitively and then started pressing into the therapist's arm around a scar with her thumbs. When asked what she was doing Philippa replied, " Making your arm better like you do mine".

Andrew is a 35 year old man who has severe learning difficulties. He has frequent epileptic fits and poor posture. He requires the assistance of at least one person to help him to walk. His circulation is sluggish and his feet and hands are constantly cold and clammy. Andrew received aromatherapy regularly at the hospital where he lived. His feet, hands and legs were massaged with essential oils which help circulatory conditions. The effect of the massage on his legs was quite startling. Instead of a bluish/white his legs became a healthy pink colour which lasted for quite some time after the massage. After an aromatherapy session Andrew is visibly more alert and requires less support when walking. He has not had any chilblains, which used to trouble him in the previous twelve months .

Belinda has congenital contractures of her feet and hips causing her to walk with great difficulty using two canes. When the massage therapist started to work with her, her feet and legs below the knees were icy cold, and her joints very sensitive to touch. Belinda was quite nervous and therefore not very relaxed. The massage therapist saw her weekly and using lavender oil in a carrier oil and apricot facial oil gently started to massage her feet, legs and face slowly and smoothly, reassuring Belinda and helping her to relax and enjoy the massage.

As Belinda became more used to it the massage therapist worked more firmly, improving the circulation back to her heart by working with firmer upward strokes on her legs, back, shoulders, neck, hands and arms. Although the massage could do little for the congenital contractures it considerably improved her circulation and eased her joints. Staff at her flat were particularly amazed at how warm her feet and legs had become. Belinda was also more relaxed in herself, and more comfortable and less nervous when doing her physiotherapy exercises.

2. To Improve Muscle Tone and Flexibility

Limbs which are not used regularly due to spasticity, contractures or other problems can lose their muscle tone and flexibility, limiting mobility and co-ordination. Regular massage combined with physiotherapy can go a long way towards improving and preparing the body for use.

Theory into Practice

Carol has Cerebral Palsy and uses a wheelchair, although she can stand and walk from room to room with support. When massage was first started her body was like a '7', bent at the hips but straight and rigid. She was massaged lying on a covered mat supported by cushions. She really enjoyed the massage and would watch as her feet and legs were massaged, smiling and lifting her feet up herself to have her shoes and socks taken off, and reaching out when she wanted an arm massaged. The staff at the day centre worked firmly on her feet, legs, hips, back, shoulders, hands, arms and neck encouraging her interest and participation and introducing physiotherapy exercises as her limbs became warmed and supple from the massage. At the end of the session (often one hour) she loved having her face massaged and would beam up at the staff and then slowly fall asleep! Regular massage increased the flexibility in her hips and back so that she could stand straighter and walk using more of her own balance and weight. Staff were amazed at how much taller she became.

Richard is a lively and talkative young man. He lives alone with his ageing father and attends an adult training centre. Five years ago he fell out of the minibus and sustained multiple fractures to one leg. Although they healed, he lost his confidence to walk and remained in a wheelchair. His physiotherapist said that although his muscles were wasted through lack of use there was no other physical reason why he should not walk again. Richard was very keen to have a go but was shaky. Being tall and large boned he was very difficult to support adequately by one person, and as his father was quite ill it was felt that the more independent Richard could be the better for himself and his carers.

The physiotherapist and one of the day centre officers started regular physiotherapy and massage on his feet, ankles, legs and back. Richard took great pride and interest in it, bringing a tracksuit each day and proudly showing how he could stand up from the wheelchair at the table. As the muscle tone and circulation improved in Richard's lower body so his shakiness reduced and his confidence increased. One year later, he could walk slowly but surely around the day centre with the support of one person and was enthusiastically trying a few steps alone. He could move himself round a room quite easily and could take himself to the toilet.

3. To Improve Digestion, Assimilation and Elimination

People who are not able to exercise or move around very much, for example people who use wheelchairs, are often prone to constipation and reliant on medication or enemas to eliminate waste. High fibre diets and massage to the lower back and abdomen can help the colon work more comfortably and naturally.

Theory into Practice

Alan uses a wheelchair all the time and is overweight. He becomes constipated and often became very bad tempered after lunch at the day centre. The staff suspected that the bad temper might be due to discomfort because of his constipation and started to massage his abdomen regularly. They did this by firmly massaging his lower back and by using gentle strokes in a clockwise direction around his abdomen. He started to go to the toilet more regularly and became less distressed after lunch.

4. To Reduce Symptoms Related to Tension

The physical symptoms of tension such as headaches or tightness in the shoulders can be greatly relieved through massage. As muscles tighten through stress they can become knotted and sore, giving great discomfort and leading to unhealthy postures such as hunched shoulders. Massage eases away the tension and improves the health of the muscles. After a good neck and shoulder massage people often comment that they feel *"a good few inches taller!"*.

Aromatherapy Recipes

The following combinations and proportions of essential oils can be used in the bath, in compresses, can be vaporised or used in 3 teaspoonsful of carrier oil or lotion for massage or application.

Aches and Pains

Chamomile *1 drop*
Lavender *2 drops*
Marjoram *1 drop*
Rosemary *1 drop*

Eucalyptus *1 drop*
Juniper *1 drop*
Lavender *1 drop*
Rosemary *2 drops*

For foot bath :
Chamomile *1 drop*
Eucalyptus *2 drops*
Juniper *1 drop*
Lavender *2 drops*

Bronchitis and Catarrh

Eucalyptus *2 drops*
Lavender *2 drops*
Peppermint *1 drop*
Sandalwood *1 drop*

Cedarwood *3 drops*
Marjoram *1 drop*
Peppermint *2 drops*

Cellulite

Cypress *1 drop*
Juniper *2 drops*
Rosemary *2 drops*

Cellulite (continued)

Geranium	*3 drops*
Juniper	*2 drops*
Lavender	*1 drop*

Detoxifying

Geranium	*2 drops*
Juniper	*2 drops*
Lavender	*1 drop*
Geranium	*2 drops*
Juniper	*2 drops*
Rosemary	*1 drop*

Poor Circulation

Juniper	*3 drops*
Rosemary	*3 drops*

Relieve cold symptoms

Eucalyptus	*2 drops*
Lavender	*1 drop*
Tea tree	*1 drop*
Rosemary	*1 drop*

Rheumatism

Juniper	*2 drops*
Lavender	*2 drops*
Marjoram	*2 drops*
Eucalyptus	*1 drop*
Juniper	*2 drops*
Rosemary	*3 drops*

Thrush

Lavender	*3 drops*
Tea tree	*3 drops*

■ The Therapeutic Index

The Therapeutic Index contains many common conditions and for each one it recommends four different essential oils which could help. It is based on sixteen of the most commonly used essential oils which were described in Chapter 6. For those who have a more extensive collection of essential oils, an additional oil is recommended in brackets for each condition.

The Therapeutic Index

Circulatory Conditions		**Methods of Use**
High blood pressure	Lavender, Lemon, Marjoram, Ylang Ylang	Bath, Inhalation, Massage, Vaporisation
Poor circulation	Cypress, Juniper, Lemon, Rosemary, (Ginger)	Bath, Massage
Varicose veins	Cypress, Lemon, Peppermint, (Neroli)	Compress, Massage
Digestive Conditions		
Appetite loss	Bergamot, Chamomile, Lemon, (Black Pepper)	Bath, Inhalation, Massage, Vaporisation
Constipation	Chamomile, Marjoram, Rosemary, (Black Pepper)	Bath, Compress, Massage
Diarrhoea	Geranium, Lavender, Lemon, Peppermint	Bath, Compress ,Massage
Flatulence	Bergamot, Peppermint, Rosemary, (Caraway)	Compress, Massage
Indigestion	Bergamot, Chamomile, Lavender, Peppermint, (Black Pepper)	Compress, Massage
Nausea & Vomiting	Chamomile, Lavender, Peppermint, Sandalwood, (Rose Otto)	Bath, Inhalation, Massage, Vaporisation
Excretory Conditions		
Cystitis	Bergamot, Juniper, Sandalwood, Tea Tree, (Black Pepper)	Bath, Massage
Fluid retention	Cypress, Eucalyptus, Juniper, (Fennel)	Bath, Compress, Massage
Haemorrhoids	Chamomile, Cypress, Juniper	Application, Bath
Urinary infections	Eucalyptus, Geranium, Juniper, Sandalwood, (Pine)	Bath, Massage
General Conditions		
Anxiety/Stress	Bergamot, Cedarwood, Chamomile, Clary Sage, Cypress, Geranium, Juniper, Lavender, Marjoram, Sandalwood, Ylang	Bath, Inhalation, Massage, Vaporisation
Burns/Wounds (minor)	Lavender, Tea Tree	Application, Compress
Depression	Bergamot, Chamomile, Clary Sage, Geranium, Lavender, Sandalwood, Ylang Ylang	Bath, Inhalation, Massage, Vaporisation
Earache	Bergamot, Chamomile, Lavender, Peppermint	Compress
Headache	Eucalyptus, Lavender, Peppermint, Rosemary	Compress , Inhalation, Massage, Vaporisation
Immune deficiency	Bergamot, Lavender, Lemon, Tea tree, (Rose Otto)	Bath, Gargle, Inhalation, Massage, Vaporisation
Insomnia	Chamomile, Juniper, Lavender, Marjoram, Sandalwood, Ylang Ylang	Bath, Inhalation, Massage, Vaporisation

Lethargy	Eucalyptus, Lemon, Peppermint, Rosemary	Bath, Inhalation, Massage, Vaporisation
Scars	Lavender, (Frankincense)	Application
Menstrual Conditions		
Heavy periods	Chamomile, Cypress, Geranium, (Rose Otto)	Bath, Compress, Massage
Irregular periods	Chamomile, Clary sage, Juniper, Lavender, (Rose Otto)	Bath, Compress, Massage
Painful periods	Chamomile, Camphor, Lavender, Marjoram, (Cajuput)	Bath, Compress, Massage
Pre-menstrual tension	Chamomile, Clary sage, Geranium, Lavender, (Neroli)	Bath, Inhalation, Massage, Vaporisation
Muscular / Skeletal Conditions		
Aches and Pains	Eucalyptus, Marjoram, Peppermint, Rosemary	Bath, Compress, Massage
Muscle cramps	Chamomile, Cypress, Lavender, Marjoram	Bath, Compress, Massage
Rheumatoid Arthritis	Chamomile, Eucalyptus, Juniper, Rosemary	Bath, Compress, Massage
Respiratory Conditions		
Asthma	Eucalyptus, Lavender, Marjoram, Peppermint, (Cajuput)	Bath, Compress, Inhalation (not steam), Massage, Vaporisation
Bronchitis	Cedarwood, Eucalyptus, Rosemary, Sandalwood, (Pine)	Bath, Compress, Gargle, Inhalation, Massage, Vaporisation
Cold	Eucalyptus, Lemon, Rosemary, Tea Tree, (Black Pepper)	Bath, Gargle, Inhalation, Vaporisation
Cough	Cedarwood, Eucalyptus, Lavender, Peppermint, (Frankincense)	Compress, Gargle, Inhalation, Vaporisation
Flu	Eucalyptus, Geranium, Rosemary	Compress, Inhalation, Vaporisation
Sinus problems	Eucalyptus, Lavender, Lemon, Peppermint, (Pine)	Bath, Inhalation, Massage, Vaporisation
Sore throat	Clary-sage, Geranium, Lavender	Compress, Gargle, Inhalation, Vaporisation
Skin Conditions		
Acne	Chamomile, Juniper, Lavender, Tea Tree, (Petitgrain)	Compress, Massage
Cellulite	Geranium, Juniper, Lavender, Rosemary, (Fennel)	Bath, Compress, Massage
Dermatitis/Eczema	Bergamot, Chamomile, Geranium, Lavender	Compress, Massage
Dry Skin	Chamomile, Geranium, Lavender, Sandalwood, (Rose Otto)	Compress, Massage
Inflamed/Sensitive	Chamomile, Clary sage, Geranium, Lavender, (Neroli)	Compress, Massage
Oily Skin	Bergamot, Cedarwood, Cypress, Lemon	Compress, Massage
Stretch marks	Lavender, (Frankincense)	Application, Compress

13

Contra-indications - The Safe Use of Essential Oils

In general, aromatherapy and massage are beneficial for most conditions. However, there are certain conditions for which massage or the use of essential oils is contra-indicated, that is, they should not be used at all, or should be used with caution.

The following information explains:

when aromatherapy and massage should be avoided completely.
when massage can be used but certain essential oils should be avoided.
which conditions are contra-indicated by massage but can be helped by using essential oils.

■ General Principles

a Do not take essential oils by mouth.

b Do not apply neat essential oils directly onto the skin. Always dilute first into a carrier of carrier oil or lotion (application, massage), water (bath, compress) or air (vaporiser, inhalations). The only exception to this rule is as an emergency measure when a tiny amount of either lavender or tea tree essential oil could be used on a sting, small burn or tiny wound.

c At least two hours should elapse after a person has eaten before they receive a full body massage.

d Seek medical advice if the person is receiving specialised treatment, or if you have any doubts. Do not massage the area surrounding a recent injection (for example, if people are receiving medication through depot injections).

e When massaging always look for any signs of discomfort such as changes in breathing, facial expression, colour or sweating.

Emergency Measures

If someone accidentally gets any essential oil or massage oil in the eye or eye area, wash thoroughly with cold clean water for 5 minutes. A drop of carrier oil into the eye will quickly dilute any neat essential oil before rinsing. If after 15 minutes the stinging has not subsided, seek medical attention.

Should a large amount of neat essential oil be spilt on a person's skin, then the area should be rinsed immediately with water. This does not apply to the very small amounts of lavender or tea tree deliberately applied as an emergency treatment for stings, bites, small cuts or burns.

Asthma

Asthma can respond very well to aromatherapy, in inhalation from a handkerchief, using essential oils in massage, in vaporisation in the room and also when used in the bath. However, inhaling the steam from a basin of hot water and essential oils, is contra-indicated as it could have the reverse effect and make breathing more difficult. The essential oils evaporate more quickly due to the heat and this extra strength, together with the steam itself, may affect the lungs.

Brittle Bones

Massage very gently and carefully.

Cancer

Unless advised otherwise by a doctor massage should not be used if a person has been diagnosed as having cancer. If a person is in the terminal stages of the illness, massage with essential oils can be used to soothe and relax.

Epilepsy

Some essential oils are thought to stimulate an epileptic fit in people who have epilepsy and should be avoided. These oils are: aniseed, dill, fennel, hyssop and sage. Many people with learning difficulties have epilepsy and some aromatherapy books suggest that rosemary is a contra-indicated oil. Pierre Franchomme, an acknowledged expert on essential oils in France, does not include any of the three varieties of rosmarinus officinalis in his list of contra-indicated oils for epilepsy. Present research suggests that rosemary is a beneficial anti-convulsive when used in low dilutions (2%) (I.J.A. Vol. 3, No. 3).

An important factor in the use of essential oils is the dosage, and excessive concentrations may well be harmful. For example, digitalis in minute amounts is very helpful in heart conditions, whereas in large amounts it can be lethal. Similarly, juniper, which is an excellent kidney stimulant in low concentrations, can overstimulate the kidney and cause toxicity if used in excessive amounts. The quantities quoted in this book have been carefully monitored and are well within safety limits.

When massaging a person who has epilepsy use slow, smooth and relaxing strokes. If in doubt contact the person's G.P.

Fractures

If fractures have been treated, it is beneficial to massage one joint above the area of the break. After the plaster cast is removed, gentle massage with essential oils can aid healing.

Heart and Circulatory Conditions

If the person has a history of heart attacks, angina or strokes use gentle massage which will help the circulation.

High Blood Pressure

For people with high blood pressure, gentle massage using relaxing essential oils is beneficial. The following stimulating essential oils should not be used for or by people with high blood pressure: hyssop, rosemary, sage and thyme.

High Temperature

If a person has a high temperature, do not give her a massage. When her temperature is back to normal, massage may be useful unless the illness is more serious than 'flu, in which case a full recovery must be made before any massage can be given. However, in some cases where it is desired to reduce temperature, and certainly for high temperature due to colds and 'flu, a bath with cooling essential oils can be very helpful. Peppermint is excellent for reducing temperature either using two or three drops of essential oil in the bath or taking peppermint herbal teas. Care must be taken when using peppermint oil in the bath as more than 2 drops may irritate the skin.

Infectious Diseases

Do not massage. For localised infections such as a sore throat, chest and behind the ears, the application of essential oils in a carrier oil on the neck can be very helpful.

Inflamed Joints

With conditions such as gout or rheumatoid arthritis, the use of massage and aromatherapy one joint above the affected area can be very beneficial to improve circulation. For example massage a person's forearm to relieve pain and stiffness in the hands and fingers.

Gentle, regular application of compresses with appropriate essential oils is also very beneficial (see Therapeutic Index).

Nervous Tension

If a person is stressed or very nervous never give an invigorating massage with brisk, quick, patting or tapping movements. For full benefit the normal aromatherapy massage with soothing, firm and even strokes, using relaxing essential oils, should be given.

Obesity / Overweight

Massage is very useful to help the circulation, in particular the return of the blood to the heart (venous return). Although the massage should be firm, avoid deep or invigorating massage with obese people as this may overtax the heart. Consideration should be given to the person's body image, helping to promote positive feelings about her body.

Pregnancy

Aromatherapy has been shown to be very helpful during pregnancy, with all its possible associated effects of heartburn, indigestion, backache and morning sickness. Invigorating and deep massage to the abdomen should be avoided.

There have not been any recorded cases of miscarriage through the use of essential oils in massage, compresses, baths or inhalation. However, in order to err on the side of safety, it is recommended that the following essential oils are avoided during pregnancy because of their possible neuro-toxic effects: basil, hyssop, sage and thyme.

In addition, the following oils should be avoided during the first 4 months of pregnancy because of their possible emmenagoguic or diuretic effects: clary sage, fennel, juniper, marjoram, rosemary and true melissa.

Scar Tissue

Avoid massaging scar tissue that is new, still red, painful, inflamed or hot. Compresses or sprays are very soothing at this stage. Massage with essential oils is beneficial for normal scar tissue.

Sensitivity to Sunlight

Some of the citrus essential oils may cause a skin reaction when exposed either to strong sunlight or a sunbed straight after application, leading to redness or allergic reactions. Therefore do not use the following oils in the bath, in a compress or in a massage oil immediately before exposure to strong sunlight or using a sunbed: bergamot, lemon, lime and orange.

Some aromatherapists suggest that bergamot should not be used on people who have eczema as it sensitises the skin to sunlight, which exacerbates this condition. No-one, ill or well, should use bergamot oil immediately before going into the sun. However, if this precept is adhered to, bergamot is actually beneficial to the relief of eczema and, after one hour, is completely absorbed into the skin, making sunlight non-hazardous.

Skin Conditions

In general avoid massaging broken skin, unexplained lumps, open wounds, infected, swollen or painful areas. A compress using healing essential oils is recommended for broken skin or wounds. Bedsores respond very well to essential oils.

a Dry flaky skin - Massage with essential oils is particularly good for people who have dry skin. However in extreme cases when the flakes are big enough and deep enough to cause skin inflammation then avoid that area with massage, though compresses can be very soothing.

b Contagious skin diseases - Do not massage.

c Acne - Certain essential oils can be beneficial used in back and facial massage to clear infection and help to improve the skin (see Therapeutic Index).

d Sensitive skin/Allergic skin - Use soothing essential oils in carrier oil and lotion or application. People who have very sensitive skin or who suffer from skin allergies may find that a few essential oils could produce an unpleasant stinging sensation when used in the bath. Use only 2 drops of the following oils: basil, clove, cinnamon, fennel, lemon, lemongrass, melissa, peppermint, thyme.

Thrombosis

Avoid massage.

Varicose Veins

Treat with care and massage very gently with upward strokes only (i.e. towards the heart). Massage above the area first.

Children

The methods and examples given throughout the book can be used with confidence with children who have learning difficulties providing that a few safety precautions are adhered to. Baths and inhalations can be used to help many of the minor childhood ailments. Most children enjoy and respond well to massage. The number of drops used by any method should be half that used for an adult.

Baths

Dilute 3 drops of essential oil in either a teaspoon of full fat milk, honey, cream or a teaspoon of carrier oil before adding to the bath.

Massage

Make a weaker blend of massage oil by diluting 1 to 2 drops of essential oil per 5ml (a teaspoonful) of carrier oil, instead of the 2-3 drops used for an adult.

Inhalations

Inhalations using a bowl of hot water must be supervised at all times and given for between 1 and 5 minutes only.

Lavender and chamomile are often used with young children for their soothing and calming properties.

Caution: do not use peppermint in inhalations for children because of its high menthol content. Do not attempt to use essential oils for a baby without advice, and never give essential oils by mouth.

Toxic Oils

Do not use any essential oil unknown to you without first consulting an authority. Some possess qualities which can be dangerous if incorrectly used. Such oils are not normally available through a reputable supplier of essential oils for aromatherapy.

Summary of Contra-Indications

Condition	Massage	Essential Oils to Avoid	Comments
Asthma			Do not inhale from essential oil in hot water
Brittle bones	Massage gently		
Cancer	Do not massage except if terminal		Seek medical advice if unsure
Epilepsy	Massage gently	Aniseed, Dill, Fennel, Hyssop, Sage	Seek medical advice if unsure
Fractures	Massage gently after cast removed		
Heart and circulatory conditions	Massage gently		Seek medical advice if unsure
High blood pressure	Massage gently	Aniseed, Rosemary, Sage, Thyme	
High temperature	Do not massage		Cold peppermint tea or 2 - 3 drops of peppermint oil in the bath can help bring temperature down
Infectious disease	Do not massage		Applying appropriate oils in carrier oil over neck and chest can be beneficial
Inflamed joints	Avoid area around joint. Massage one joint above		
Nervous tension	Massage gently		

Condition	Massage	Essential Oils to Avoid	Comments
Obesity / overweight	Massage gently		Consideration should be given to person's body image
Pregnancy	Massage only very gently on the abdomen	Basil, Hyssop, Sage, Thyme. Clary sage, Fennel, Juniper, Marjoram, Melissa and Rosemary should be avoided duringthe first five months	
Scar tissue	Avoid if new, red, painful, hot or inflamed		Massage is beneficial for normal scar tissue. Compresses are soothing for new scar tissue
Sensitivity to sunlight		Bergamot, Lemon, Lime, Orange	
Skin conditions:			
Dry skin	Beneficial unless inflamed		
Contagious	Do not massage		
Sensitive		Basil, Cinnamon, Clove, Fennel, Lemon, Lemongrass, Melissa, Peppermint, Tea Tree, Thyme	
Other	Avoid broken skin, unexplained lumps, open wounds and painful, swollen or infected areas		Compress or water spray with healing essential oils for broken skin and wounds
Thrombosis	Do not massage		
Varicose veins	Massage very gently always towards the heart		First clear the area *above* a very congested vein

14

Choosing Essential Oils

There are many essential oils to choose from, some which promote relaxation and others which refresh and invigorate. In this chapter we will consider how to help the individual choose oils simply to relax or invigorate. We will also explain how to choose essential oils to improve a person's health.

■ Choosing Relaxing or Invigorating oils

If you simply want to help a person to relax using a pleasant fragrance, then choosing which oils to use is relatively simple. From the relaxing oils suggested, the best ones to use would be the person's favourites. It is advisable not to present all the relaxing oils at once, as at best the nose can only cope with 3 to 4 different smells in succession. A good way would be to choose 3 different essential oils and encourage the person to smell each one for a couple of seconds. Choose perhaps a floral essence such as lavender, and contrast this with a citrus aroma such as bergamot and a woody fragrance such as sandalwood. If the person appears to prefer the floral aroma, then in another session you could offer 3 different floral fragrances such as lavender, ylang ylang and geranium.

Once the favourite has been established, for example lavender, it could then be used on its own or in combination with another oil which the person likes. If the person has difficulty in sleeping, offer her the more sedative oils to choose from which include:

Chamomile
Juniper
Lavender
Marjoram
Sandalwood
Ylang ylang

If the person wants to relax and yet be uplifted at the same time choose from bergamot, clary sage, geranium, or lavender. Use the same principle if the person wants to be invigorated or to improve her concentration. Discover the person's favourite from the invigorating oils of eucalyptus, lemon, peppermint or rosemary and use them in either the bath, a vigorous massage or a vaporiser. This is the best way to begin selecting oils for those with learning difficulties, though do try adding a second oil for extra effect once one has been established. For further ways of selection, training in aromatherapy is necessary.

Choosing Essential Oils to Help Minor Health Problems

The Therapeutic Index can be used as a guide if you want to use essential oils to help a specific health problem. If the person has skin problems such as acne, turn to the index and look up the oils which are recommended for that condition. These are lavender, chamomile, juniper and tea tree. You could use the 4 oils suggested in combination, or simply ask the person which she prefers and mix those together. The recipe section is a guide to the combinations and quantities which have been found to be useful. The oils could either be added to a carrier oil, used in the bath, or in a compress as indicated in the methods section.

If you want to help the person primarily to relax, but you are also interested in helping her aches and pains, then look at the oils recommended for aches and pains and cross reference these with the list of relaxing oils. Are any of those oils which are recommended for aches and pains also oils for relaxing? If so, select that oil or oils. As well as helping the person to relax, you will also be helping her aches and pains. If there is only one common oil, and you want to use more than one, use the one which appears in both lists, plus any other oil from the relaxing range.

A professional aromatherapist may employ several different methods when choosing which oils to use. She would make a comprehensive holistic analysis, including finding out about the person's medical background, lifestyle, sleeping patterns, diet, work and stress level. An examination of the person's reflex points on the foot may follow. Along with this information she may also use other methods to help to choose the most appropriate oil, including chemical composition, muscle testing, scientific dowsing or intuition, based on a sound knowledge of essential oils.

■ Summary

To help a person to relax, to sleep, to be invigorated or uplifted, use the relevant oils in chapters 8 and 9.

To help a minor health condition

Look up the problem and choose the person's favourites from those oils which are recommended (see Therapeutic Index).

To relax/invigorate whilst helping a minor health condition

Look up the problem and cross reference the oils recommended with the list of relaxing/invigorating oils. Choose the oil which is a relaxing/invigorating oil, yet also features on the list of recommended oils for that problem.

Here are a few examples to clarify this process of choosing essential oils to relax or invigorate, whilst taking into account any specific minor health problems.

These examples are hypothetical and concentrate on the person's needs rather than presenting a balanced picture of her strengths as well as her needs.

■ Example Number One

Background

You support a young woman who has severe learning difficulties and lives in her own home in the community. She generally appears quite agitated and nervous. Sometimes she pinches the skin on her arms and that of the support staff when she is upset. Just before menstruation she appears to become very agitated and the incidence of pinching increases.

Comment

From this brief pen portrait it is possible to identify areas in which aromatherapy and massage could help. Note that the incidence of pinching seems to increase just before menstruation, suggesting that it could possibly be linked to pre-menstrual tension (P.M.T.). To identify whether this is the case it may be necessary to work with a psychologist and other support staff to record exactly when the incidences of pinching take place to identify whether there is a definite pattern of pinching before menstruation. If the woman does suffer from P.M.T., then a nutritional supplement of evening primrose oil could help.

Aim

The aim of using aromatherapy and massage would be to help this person to relax using an oil or oils which could also help P.M.T.

Contra-indications

It is necessary to check whether there are any other health considerations or contra-indications which need to be taken into account. Does she suffer from any of the contra-indications listed (Chapter 13), for example sensitive/allergic skin, high blood pressure, epilepsy?

Choosing Essential Oils

To identify which oils are relaxing and which oils could help P.M.T. it is useful to list them all and then cross reference them.

Relaxing oils:

Bergamot	*Juniper*
Cedarwood	*Lavender*
Chamomile	*Marjoram*
Clary Sage	*Sandalwood*
Cypress	*Ylang Ylang*
Geranium	

From the Therapeutic Index the following list of oils for P.M.T. is given:

Chamomile	*Geranium*
Clary Sage	*Lavender*

Each of the 4 essential oils given for P.M.T. are also relaxing oils and therefore any would be suitable. A combination of all 4 could be used, or each offered to the person for her to identify which is her favourite, and that particular oil used on its own. As the oils are synergistic (working better in combination), a mixture of 2 or more of these oils would be better.

Essential oils chosen:

Chamomile	*Geranium*
Clary Sage	*Lavender*

Carrier oil chosen:

Grapeseed

If you want to make a massage oil which would last for a few months, 5ml of wheatgerm should be added to 95ml of grapeseed oil. An extra 5ml of avocado oil added to the carrier oil would increase its penetrative powers. Another specialised carrier oil is that of evening primrose, which could be added to the grapeseed as well as, or instead of, the avocado oil, as it is known for its ability to help P.M.T.

Methods

Massage

The massage oil could be used for regular hand, foot, facial or back massage at home. A local aromatherapist or massage therapist could possibly be found to give regular full body massage.

Bath

6 drops of either geranium, clary sage, lavender or chamomile could be used in the bath. Alternatively, and more effective, would be 2 drops each of 2 of the oils or a combination of 1 drop of each.

Vaporise

Any of the 4 oils, either singly or in combination could be vaporised to give calming and relaxing ambience. The oils could be vaporised using a burner, vaporising ring, or a saucer of water on a radiator. It could be done at any time of the day, particularly when the person appears anxious or agitated.

■ Example Number Two

Background

You are supporting a 42 year old man who lives in a hostel. He regularly suffers from colds which affect his sinuses badly. He has difficulty getting to sleep, but once asleep has difficulty waking up in the morning and is often late for the adult training centre.

Comment

As he regularly suffers from colds it is likely that he has a poor immune system. Working closely with people at the training centre and living with lots of other people in close proximity often means that viruses and bacterial infections can get passed from one person to another very quickly. Odourless garlic capsules have been found to help the immune system, and it is important to ensure that this person is getting enough Vitamin C.

Aim

The aim of using aromatherapy and massage would be to help him to relax and sleep at night and invigorate him in the morning using oils to boost the immune system.

Contra-indications

Check that he is not suffering from any contra-indications, for example high blood pressure, epilepsy or sensitive skin. If not, the oils chosen will be based on those which strengthen the immune system, also bearing in mind when to use the relaxing oils and when to use the invigorating ones.

Choosing Essential Oils

In order to choose oils which can invigorate, oils which can relax and oils which can strengthen the immune system it is helpful to list the relevant oils:

Relaxing and sedative oils:

Chamomile
Juniper
Lavender
Marjoram
Sandalwood
Ylang Ylang

Invigorating oils:

Eucalyptus
Bergamot
Lemon
Peppermint
Rosemary

Immuno-strengthening oils:

Bergamot
Chamomile
Lavender
Lemon

Lemon and bergamot essential oils can invigorate and also strengthen the immune system; lavender and chamomile will also strengthen it and yet be relaxing and sedative.

Essential oils chosen:

Lemon and bergamot -	*To invigorate and strengthen the immune system.*
Lavender and chamomile -	*To relax and strengthen the immune system.*

Carrier oil chosen:

Grapeseed plus 5% wheatgerm, 5% avocado (for example, 90ml of grapeseed with 5ml of wheatgerm and 5ml of avocado added to it).

Method

Evening
When he needs to relax in the evening before going to bed, 4 drops of lavender and 2 drops of chamomile can be added to the bath water. A gentle massage could be given if he wishes, using a massage oil made from these oils in a grapeseed carrier. A few drops of lavender or chamomile oil under the pillow slip could also help to promote a peaceful sleep.

Morning
4 drops of lemon and 2 drops of bergamot in the bath would be a good start to the day, and lemon vaporised in the bedroom would help him to get going in the morning. If he catches a cold which affects his sinuses then use 4 drops of eucalyptus and 2 drops of lemon. If his sinuses are particularly troublesome then inhaling oils for sinus problems over a bowl of hot water should ease his breathing.

To help to prevent the spread of colds both at the adult training centre and the hostel, vaporise bactericidal and anti-viral oils such as pine, lavender and tea tree. Put a couple of drops of eucalyptus inside the pillow slip to ease his breathing at night.

■ Example Number Three

Background

You work with a woman who has severe learning difficulties and has lived in a large institution all her life. In six months she will be resettled into a home of her own. The skin on her arms is red and dry, and she continually scratches it. The Doctor has diagnosed mild eczema. She has epilepsy. Being full of nervous energy, she talks very quickly and is rarely still. You have noticed that her hands and feet are always cold and tend to be white in winter.

Comment

Eczema is very often stress related, so using relaxing oils may also indirectly help her eczema. Cold hands and feet suggest poor circulation, which can be helped by regular massage using essential oils.

Aim

The aim of using aromatherapy and massage is to help the person to relax using oils which could help her eczema and poor circulation.

Contra-indications

The woman suffers from two conditions for which some essential oils are contra-indicated. As she has eczema, it may be better to avoid oils which irritate sensitive skin. These are lemongrass, basil, melissa, lemon, peppermint, thyme and fennel. The fact that she has epilepsy means that oils of sage, aniseed, fennel, dill and hyssop should not be used either.

Choosing Essential Oils

We need to consider oils which are relaxing and could also help poor circulation and eczema.

Relaxing oils:

Bergamot	*Juniper*
Cedarwood	*Lavender*
Chamomile	*Marjoram*
Clary sage	*Sandalwood*
Cypress	*Ylang ylang*
Geranium	

Oils for eczema:

Bergamot	*Juniper*
Chamomile	*Geranium*

Oils for poor circulation:

Cypress	*Lemon*
Juniper	*Rosemary*

Juniper is one essential oil which is helpful for all these conditions. All the essential oils suggested for eczema are relaxing, and any could be used according to the person's preference. A good overall choice would be cypress and juniper, together with any 2 of the oils for relaxation and eczema.

Essential oils chosen:

Cypress	*Geranium*
Chamomile	*Juniper*

Carrier oil chosen:

Grapeseed with 5% wheatgerm, 5% avocado added (for example, 90ml of grapeseed oil with 5ml of wheatgerm and 5ml of avocado).

Method

Massage

Regular hand and foot massage with the massage oil given above should help to improve the condition of her skin. By using a portable foot spa with 4 drops of the oils for poor circulation, and then using the massage oil the circulation in her feet will be stimulated.

Bath

Chamomile, geranium and juniper either singly or together with cypress will provide a very soothing and relaxing bath.

Vaporisation

The person could choose between bergamot, chamomile, geranium and lavender to be used in a burner, air spray or in a saucer of water to give a calm and soothing atmosphere.

■ Example Number Four

Background

You work as a teacher in a Special School with children who have learning difficulties. One eight year old boy in your group has stiff hands and fingers which he has difficulty using. This stiffness subsides temporarily after his weekly physiotherapy session. The child also has difficulty concentrating in some classes and sometimes falls asleep. His mother complains that he does not sleep well at night.

Comments

Massage with relaxing and uplifting oils can help to relax and release stiff joints. Discuss with the physiotherapist the possibility of using hand massage regularly to help the boy to be able to increase the mobility in his hands and ask her whether she thinks there are any contra-indications to this. It is important to consult a physiotherapist wherever possible, whilst acknowledging that she may not have the time to do the daily massage herself. It would be useful to discuss with his mother the possibility of using relaxing and sedative essential oils at night to encourage sleep, helping the boy to get a good night's rest and thus help him to stay awake during class. The physiotherapist may be able to teach his mother, the teacher and any relevant care staff a simple hand massage.

Aim

To use aromatherapy and massage to help the boy to relax his hands giving increased movement, and to use oils that could help him to sleep at night and concentrate during the day.

Contra-indications

The child does not suffer from any condition for which essential oils are contra-indicated.

Choosing the Essential Oils

Relaxing and Uplifting essential oils:

Bergamot	*Geranium*
Clary sage	*Lavender*

Sedative essential oils:

Chamomile	*Marjoram*
Juniper	*Sandalwood*
Lavender	*Ylang ylang*

Invigorating essential oils:

Eucalyptus	*Peppermint*
Lemon	*Rosemary*

Give the boy an opportunity to choose his favourite essential oil(s) from the list of relaxing and uplifting oils as these may help to relax his fingers as well as being refreshing to use in a massage oil for his hands. Allow him to choose 2 of the sedative oils listed above for his mother to use with him at home. From the list of invigorating oils allow him to choose which he prefers to go with rosemary, which is one of the best oils for concentration.

Methods

At School

Use his favourite relaxing oil in a grapeseed carrier base for regular daily hand massage prior to using his hands in another activity.

His favourite invigorating oil could be vaporised with rosemary using a vaporising ring in the class room to help both him and his classmates to concentrate.

At Home

Use his favourite sedative oils in an evening bath, using 4 drops of oil in total diluted in a teaspoonful of carrier oil, perhaps followed by a relaxing foot massage using the same mix.

Vaporise a sedative oil in the bedroom prior to bedtime and use a couple of drops of lavender or another sedative oil inside the pillow slip to promote a restful and peaceful night's sleep.

15

Creating a Relaxing and Supportive Environment

There are many different ways of using massage. It can be used on a one-to-one basis or with a small group, for a few minutes or up to one hour. Whichever way you choose, there are some basic principles to consider which will help to ensure that the person is able to relax and benefit from the massage as much as possible.

Preparing the Area

Temperature

The room should be warm and preferably draught free. As the person relaxes she may become more sensitive to coolness; warmth helps to promote relaxation and is also comforting. After a massage always air the room thoroughly.

Lighting

Lighting is important. Bright lights and particularly fluorescent lights are intrusive. Soft lighting is preferable.

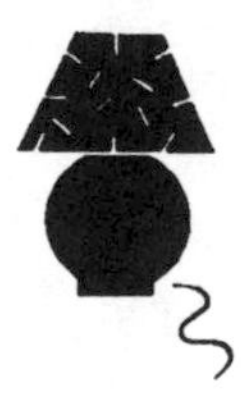

Comfort

The person being massaged needs to be comfortable. If she is lying on a carpeted floor then you may only need a blanket or sleeping bag underneath to give some support. However if the floor is hard then a mat, foam mattress or soft bean bag is better, covered with towels and with a pillow or cushion to support the head. If the person has physical disabilities you may find that more cushions are required to give additional support. For a full body massage

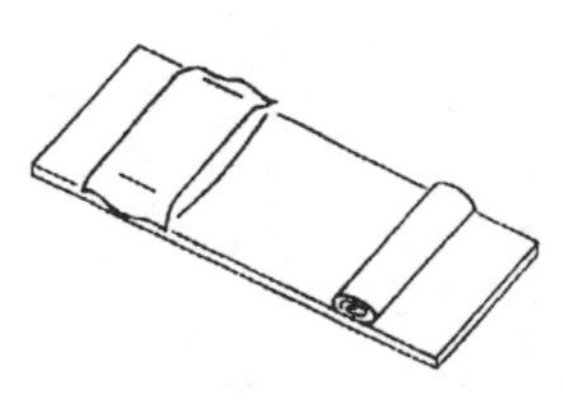

the floor or a massage couch is better than a bed, which may be soft, making it difficult to keep the pressure even. It also makes it easier to look after yourself, reducing the likelihood of backache through awkward postures. Beds can be difficult to get around, reach across and bend over. A portable massage couch is better, but its height may make it unsafe for some people with severe learning difficulties and multiple disabilities. Some firms, however, can supply couches to any specifications.

Noise

Ideally the time given for massage should be quiet and undisturbed. This may be difficult in a busy unit, but interruptions should be kept to a minimum. A side room is better than a busy activities room and a bedroom may be more conducive than a living room.

Massage environment

It helps if the room itself is pleasant to be in. Plants help to enhance a room and if you want to experiment with colour schemes and/or coloured lighting, the following may serve as a guide:

The blue shades are particularly good for massage, being calm, gentle and generally more positive colours. For example blue and turquoise can reduce tension and sleeplessness making a room feel fresh and spacious. Experiments have shown that blue light can lead to a lowering of blood pressure whilst red light can lead to an increase in blood pressure (Kirsta, A. 1986). Pink is associated with tranquillity, composure and spirituality. Violet is connected with inner balance, peace and calm.

White represents purity and spirituality. However its effect can vary from calming to cold and irritating. Many people get a 'hospital' feeling in white rooms. Green is a good colour as it represents equilibrium and lack of movement. It can induce lethargy and relaxation.

The more orange shades are not so conducive. Yellow can be irritating or give a 'spaceless' feeling. Orange in itself is joyful but can feel sticky and stifling, reducing space. Red stimulates and warms but can be oppressive. Brown shades are protective.

Aroma

To fragrance the room or to make the session more relaxing or invigorating you could vaporise essential oils.

Contact

Have everything you need close at hand. When you give a massage you need to be able to maintain contact with the person. Having oils, lotions, towels, blankets etc. at hand reduces the need to get up and break contact.

Music

Some people enjoy soft, relaxing background music whilst others find it distracting and prefer quiet.

■ Preparing Yourself

Massage is a two way activity and it is as important to prepare yourself as to prepare the person you are going to massage.

Clothing

Wear loose and comfortable clothes, bearing in mind that they may get oils and creams on them. Remove any rings, watches or jewellery that may get in the way. Preferably keep your nails short.

Focus your attention.

Massage is a wonderful form of communication but to be effective the giver must be able to focus solely on the person receiving the massage. This will be easier if you bear the following things in mind:-

How is your posture?

This obviously affects how comfortable you are. If you are massaging on the floor a comfortable position for most people is to kneel, keeping the back as straight as possible. By moving from the knees up and down you can shift your body weight to apply pressure, which is less tiring than applying pressure with your arms and from your shoulders. Remember that how you are feeling will be transmitted clearly to the person you are massaging, so if you are relaxed and comfortable it will be more reassuring for the person. If you are using a massage couch, stand with your feet apart, the front foot level with the person's hip when massaging the back. This prevents you from straining your back.

How are you feeling emotionally?

If you are feeling tense, upset, irritable or angry, those feelings will affect the quality of touch that you are able to give and will be sensed by the person you are massaging. To improve the focus of your attention try being aware of your feelings and then imagine setting them on one side, not blocked, but to be dealt with or expressed later when it is more appropriate to do so. This is a form of 'centering' and with practice can be an effective way of dealing with 'the here and now' more clearly.

How are you breathing?

Another way to help relax and focus yourself is to focus for a minute on your breathing. When we are rushed we tend to breathe quickly and into our chests. By breathing more slowly and deeply into the abdomen it is possible to relax and feel calmer. If you find that difficult to do try lying down with one hand on your abdomen and one on your chest and notice how fast you are breathing and where. Try breathing more deeply into your stomach so that the lower hand rises and falls with your breath. Notice how you feel after a while and then just let your breath flow naturally.

Preparing the Individual

Communicate your intention

As mentioned before, an important part of any activity is to communicate what you would like to do and give the person choices. Finding a way to prepare the person in this way can be a challenging but crucial part of the activity. How you communicate will depend on the abilities and disabilities of each person. If a verbal phrase such as 'shall I rub/massage your feet' is not understood try signing 'M' for massage on the person's hand and/or rub some cream or make a circling movement with the flats of your fingers on the back of the person's hand to communicate your intention. Giving people who have dual sensory impairment a particular essential oil diluted in a vegetable oil or lotion to smell becomes a familiar sign that they can associate with massage. In these ways each person can learn to recognize the sign and be given the opportunity to choose whether she would like massage at that time or not. We all have times when we would like to be touched, and times when we would not, and it is important for each person to be able to make that choice at any given moment.

Choosing oils

Take the person to the designated area and tell her again what is going to happen. Perhaps at this stage you could give her a choice between 2 or 3 different relaxing oils to smell.

Physical comfort and support

Make sure that the person is comfortable, having removed any clothing or jewellery as necessary. If she has a hearing aid make sure that you turn it off or remove it before massaging the neck and face otherwise it will whistle. If lying on her front, a pillow under the chest and support under the ankles (eg. a rolled up towel) will make her more comfortable. If lying on her back, a pillow under the head and support under the knees will help her to relax.

Individual needs

Plan the sessions to meet the person's individual requirements. For example the best time to relax somebody may be after she has had a swim, after a bath or before she goes to bed. If she has regular physiotherapy the best time for massage may be before the physiotherapy to help relax, loosen and warm her. If she finds physiotherapy stressful or tiring, a massage straight afterwards may make her more comfortable. Pay attention to details that will enhance the success of a massage session for a particular person. Use the essential oils that may help her to relax, and talk softly and reassuringly to help her feel safer, or tuck her in with warm towels to promote a sense of security and comfort.

Theory into Practice

Jill has dual sensory impairment with severe learning difficulties. She had recently been moved from a large hospital to a small residential and educational unit for adults with multiple disabilities. There had been no way of explaining to her why she was being moved, so faced with a strange environment Jill became very anxious, distressed and started crying, pulling out her hair and not sleeping.

The massage therapist started by giving Jill some oils to smell. She liked the peppermint foot lotion and lavender oil so some of the first was rubbed into the back of Jill's hand and her hands shaped into the sign for bedroom so that Jill would learn to associate the two signs together as indicating massage in her bedroom. In her room, away from other distractions, the windows were closed and the radiator put on. Towels were warmed over the radiator. The massage therapist quickly found that Jill enjoyed the massage and that when her hands were being massaged she would show great interest, moving her own fingers round and trying to 'help' the therapist. However when her feet were being massaged she would be totally still, smile, her breathing would deepen and on occasions she would fall asleep.

The first few times Jill enjoyed the massage for 10-15 minutes but then became suddenly distressed and agitated, pulling her hair violently and crying. It soon became apparent that as she relaxed she often needed to go to the toilet, so at first the session would be ended abruptly and Jill would have to be taken to the toilet. Later the staff took her to the toilet before the massage and Jill would then have her feet, legs and back massaged. Then she would be covered in warm towels and left to sleep. Jill still enjoys massage, is sleeping well and has a good trusting relationship with her key worker and the other members of staff.

16

Massage Techniques

Using Oils and Lotions

It is very difficult to give an effective massage without the use of an oil or lotion. The friction between your hands and the person's skin makes it difficult to move smoothly while applying appropriate pressure. Never pour oil directly from the bottle onto the person's skin. If you have ever had suntan lotion poured directly from the bottle onto your back, you will remember the cold, jumpy feeling it gives you. Always *briefly* rub the oil onto your own hands first. This will warm it up and lubricate your hands before making contact with the person. The use of a squeezy bottle makes it easier to regulate the amount of oil you pour out each time. Only pour out about half a teaspoon of oil into your hand at any one time. You can take more if you need to but pouring too much in the first instance will make your contact too slippery. Remember however, that a hairy body needs more oil or you will pull the hairs as you massage. Once you have made contact with the person it is best to maintain it. Make and break contact gently, only when it is absolutely necessary.

How to Use Your Hands

Most people are quite nervous about doing massage for the first time. They are worried that they may hurt the person or cause some irreparable damage. The reality is that it is difficult to hurt someone with massage and that a firm confident touch is actually more reassuring and soothing than a light nervous tickle. Here are some suggestions that may make the initial contact less daunting;

1. Keep your hands relaxed. If you are nervous the tendency will be to straighten your hands and hold them stiffly so that you apply

too much pressure with the heel of your hand or the fingertips. By relaxing your hands and keeping them loose and flexible it will be easier for you to mould the contours of the part of the body you are working on whilst keeping as much of your whole hand as possible (heel, palm and fingers) in contact with the person.

2. Look after yourself. By keeping your whole body loose and flexible, it is easy to look after rather than tire yourself or hurt your back when you are massaging. Be aware of tightening or hunching your shoulders, clenching your jaw or stooping and/or hurting your lower back. By keeping your back straight and moving at the knees or hips you protect your own back and can move more easily, using your body weight to exert pressure rather than pressing down with your arms, which strains your shoulders.

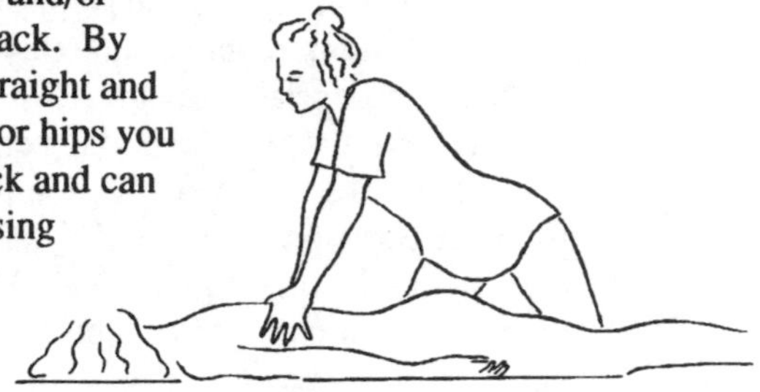

3. Use appropriate pressure. Different parts of the body will need different sorts of touch and pressure. By really feeling your way rather than gliding over or handling roughly, you will be able to gauge your touch accordingly. For example, you can work quite finely but firmly with your thumb and fingertips around the bones of the hand and wrist but use your body weight to enhance the pressure exerted through your whole hand as you work on larger areas like legs or the back.

4. Keep your strokes even. As you become more practised and comfortable with the massage try and keep your strokes even in pressure for the whole area that you are covering and build up a rhythm. The speed can vary but remember that what you do will affect the way that the person responds. If your movements are even and rhythmical it will be easier for the person to relax and 'let go'. If they are quick, uneven or interspersed with taps or tickles the person will be stimulated. That is fine if the aim of session is to invigorate the person but if you are trying to relax them then your work is undone.

5. Above all remember that whatever you do you are not just touching a part of a body, but a whole person, and even just working on one hand can have a profound and wonderful effect.

Before massaging a person with learning difficulties practice your massage on friends, family and colleagues so that you can massage with confidence.

17

Massaging the Hands and Feet

The following instructions serve as a guide for you to follow as you learn to massage. The important thing to remember is that massage is an extension of the natural urge to rub or stroke something better, so it is more important for you to feel your own way and find what feels right and comfortable, than to worry too much about technique. Remember always to explain to the person what you are doing as you begin.

■ Massaging the Hands

We use our hands so much throughout the day for doing, giving and receiving that it is easy to take them for granted. They are a wonderful part of the body to start massaging. For one thing they are easily accessible and being so sensitive can be an effective way of making contact and affecting the person. Indeed the hands, like the feet, have many reflex points which reflect different parts of the body, so hand massage can affect more than just the health of the hand. As with many types of massage, hand massage can have a variety of effects depending on your intentions. Here are just a few examples of how hand massage has been used for people who have severe learning difficulties:

1. *To promote relaxation*
2. *To promote body awareness*
3. *To relieve stiffness and pain*
4. *To break down scar tissue*
5. *To improve circulation in the hand*
6. *To help the person become accustomed to touch and manipulation of the hand (to improve tolerance of nail cutting for example)*
7. *To prepare for developing communication, for example hand signing, or through Interactive Massage.*
8. *To improve relationships and trust.*

> Through our arms and hands, we express our most powerful emotions, showing love by embracing, giving, protecting or stroking, hatred or rage through hitting, punching, shaking our fists. An arm and hand massage is thus a marvellously liberating and relaxing experience, especially for those who tend to 'bottle up' their feelings. [1]

Some parts of the hand are more sensitive than others. If the person that you are working with is nervous or wary of touch, it is best to start with the least sensitive areas. For example, it may be less threatening for the person if you start on her less dominant hand (i.e. left hand if she is right handed) and on the back of her hand rather than on her palm. If the aim of your massage is to make the person feel more relaxed and comfortable in herself or with you, then it is worth tuning into the little nuances that will make all the difference.

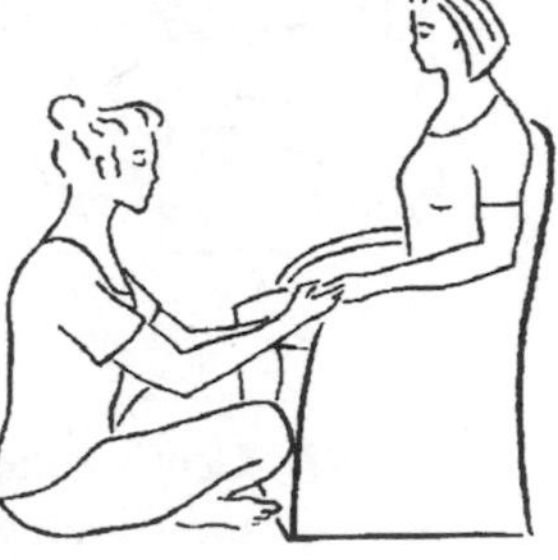

1. Make sure the person is comfortable, either lying down or sitting up, and that the arm is supported at the elbow (e.g. resting on the arm of the chair), so that the hand can be moved freely without the person having to hold it up for you.

2. Gently but firmly make some contact with the person's hand. Hold the whole hand sandwiched between your own for a few seconds or just lay one hand over the person's wrist.

3. Lift the person's hand and holding it firmly underneath with your fingers, slowly and firmly draw the heels of both your hands from the middle of the person's hand outwards. Stop when the heels of your hands are at the edge of the person's hands. Do this several times to open and stretch it.

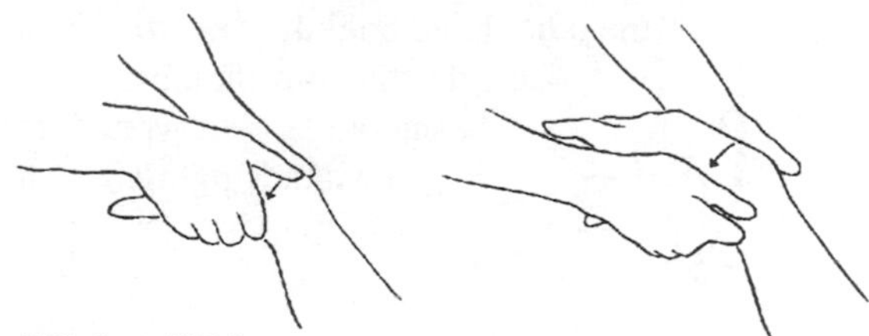

1. Clare Maxwell Hudson (1984)

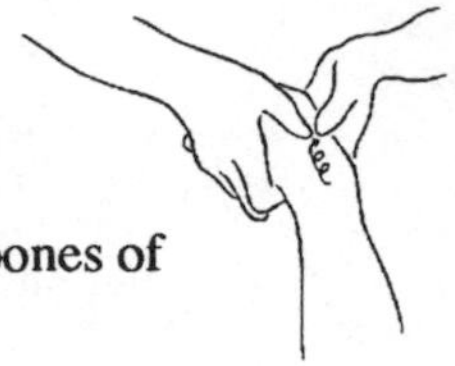

4. Now use your thumbs to work in small circles over the whole area of the back of the hand, up between the bones of the hand and around the bones of the wrist.

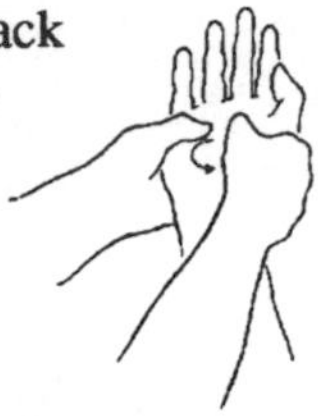

5. Turn the person's hand palm up and supporting the back of the hand this time with your fingers, massage with your thumbs in small clockwise movements over the whole palm, working all the muscles and joints and opening up the hand.

6. Now move onto the fingers. Hold the person's hand with one of yours and wrapping your whole hand or thumb and forefinger round the person's thumb, gently slide your fingers up from the base to the tip of the thumb. Pull a little as you go and twist your hand from side to side as you would opening a bottle with a corkscrew. Don't pull too hard. It is good to give the joints a gentle stretch but not to force them to crack. Do each finger in the same way.

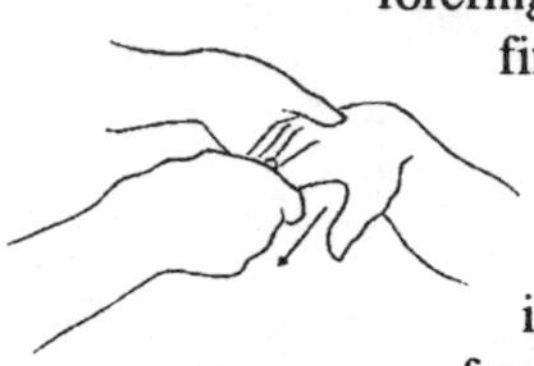

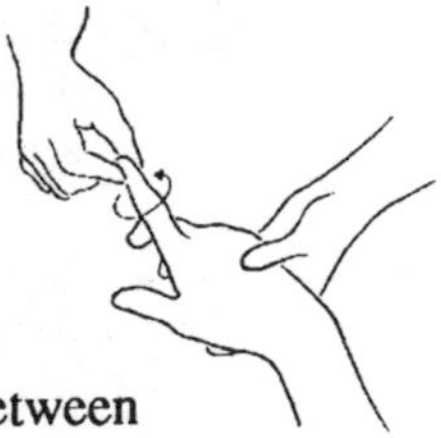

7. Gently rotate each finger. If the person finds it difficult to relax or if she wants to be helpful she may do the movement for you. If you want to help her to relax and to "let go", slow your movement or reverse the direction.

8. End by holding the person's whole hand again between both of yours. Lay it back down gently. Repeat with the other hand. It is always nice if you have time to massage both hands or both feet. You will certainly notice the difference in tension and a feeling of imbalance if you have had only one hand massaged.

9. If you want to massage the forearm as well to stimulate the circulation down to the hand, hold the hand with one of yours. With the other hand hold the arm with your fingers together down one side and your thumb the other and using long smooth strokes work firmly up the arm drawing the hands lightly down each time to start again.

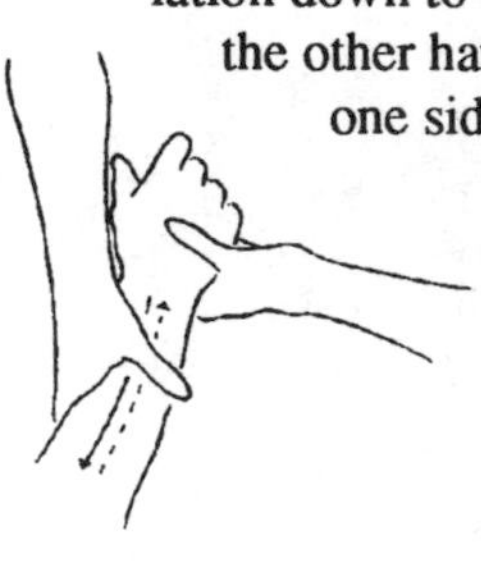

■ Massaging the Feet

Reflexology is based on the principle that there are points or areas of the feet and hands that correspond to each part of the body. By rubbing and working on these points reflexologists can improve the overall health of a person. Massaging the foot inevitably touches many of these points and a good foot massage can do much to reduce overall tension. Many of us live 'up in our heads', thinking and worrying, detached from our feet and legs. Headaches and cold feet are a clear sign that the body is out of balance. Foot massage can draw the attention down, thus helping to restore balance. Notice how quickly the feet warm up whilst massaging them.

Although foot massage will not correct deformities such as contractures it can improve the overall condition, circulation and flexibility of the foot. For people who are nervous about having their toe nails cut or seeing the chiropodist, foot massage is a pleasant way to help the person become accustomed to having her feet handled. For some individuals, their only experience of their feet being touched may be having shoes and socks put on them. If a person has poor circulation, her awareness of her feet may be diminished. Using massage and essential oils, after using a foot spa and drying the feet with a warm fluffy towel, the feet may be appreciated in a different way. The strokes for the feet are very similar to those for the hand. You may find that a carrier lotion with added essential oils gives a smoother movement than a carrier oil.

1. Make sure the person is comfortable, either sitting up or, preferably, lying down. Make sure that the person can relax her foot and does not have to hold it up for you. Prop it upon a cushion or on your own leg.

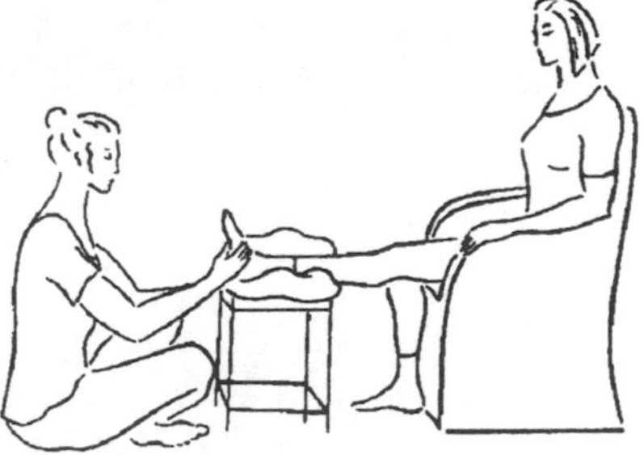

2. Make some contact. Lay one hand over the person's foot or sandwich the foot between your hands.

3. Holding the foot between the hands stroke firmly up the foot several times from the toes to the heel and ankle.

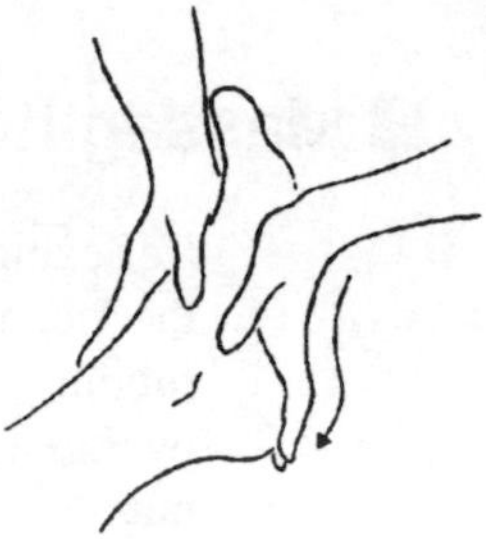

4. Then hold it firmly underneath with your fingers and use the heels of your hands to open and stretch the top of the foot from the middle outwards.

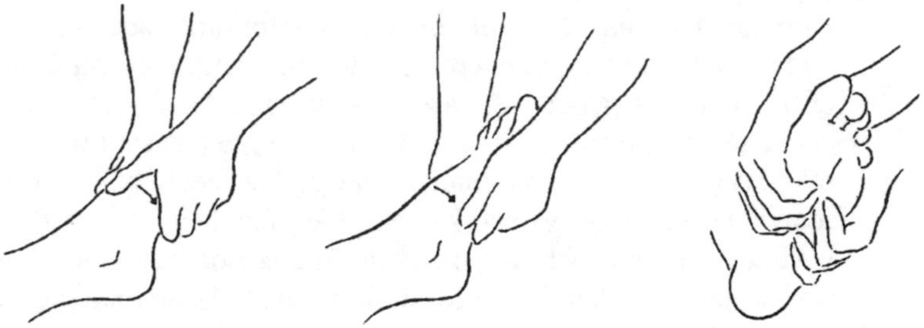

5. Holding the foot with your fingers, go over the top of the foot with your thumbs working in small circular movements. Make sure you cover the whole area slowly and thoroughly.

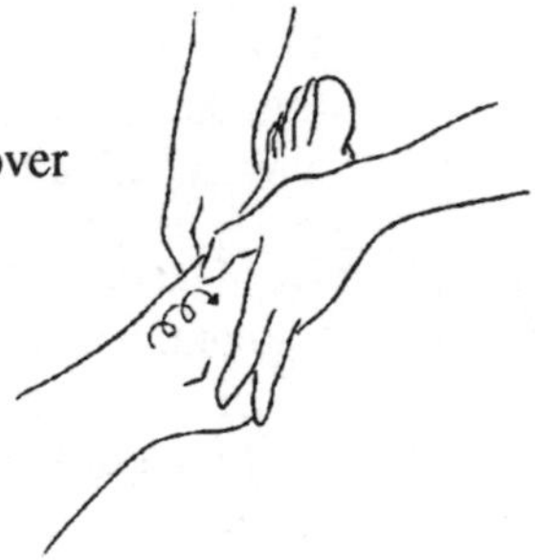

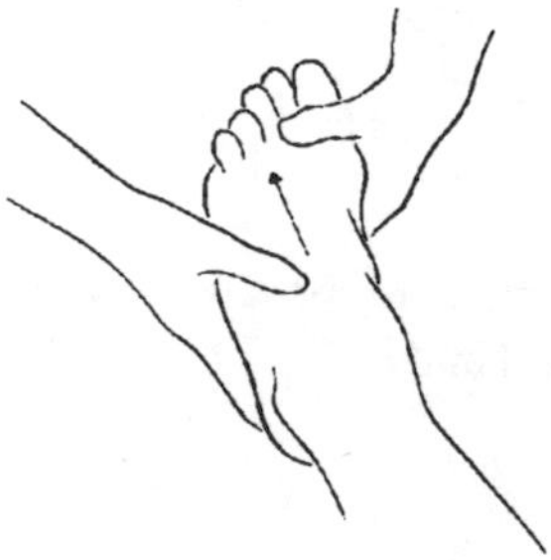

6. Draw your thumb up once along each valley between the tendons that run from the ankle to the toes.

7. Next work over the sole of the foot using your thumbs in the same way. You may find some hard crystal-like areas. They may be a little tender to work on but are an indication that that particular reflex point is blocked. Sometimes these blocks may be easily alleviated but don't overwork points that are very tender. They may reflect quite a chronic area of ill-health, better left to a qualified reflexologist. Again, cover the whole area.

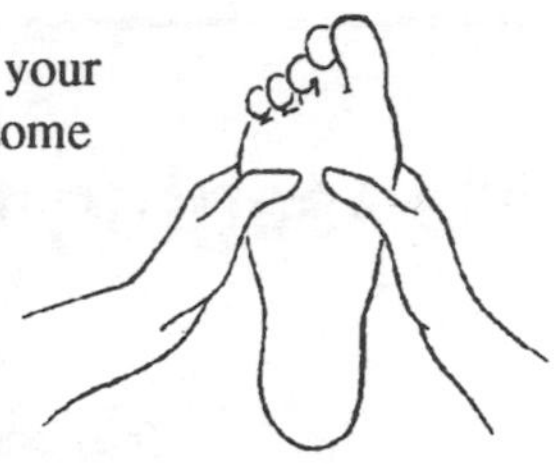

8. When you reach the heel, gently lift it up and work all around the heel with your thumbs and fingertips.

9. Lay the foot down and circle the ankle bone itself on either side of the ankle. Circle it several times with your finger tips. Go gently if this is tender for the person.

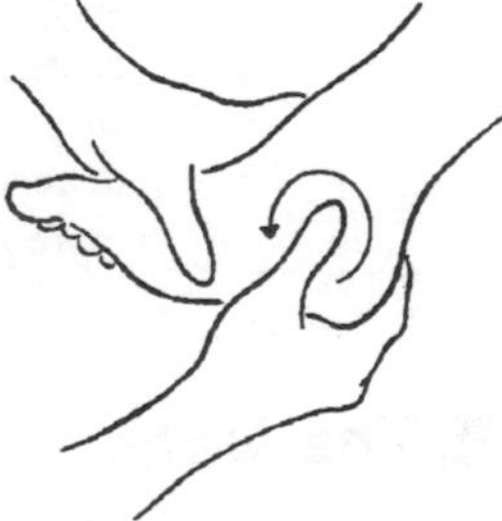

10. Now onto the toes. As with the fingers, slide your wrapped hand or finger and thumb from the base to the tip of each one pulling gently as you go.

11. Gently rotate each toe holding it at the tip. Rotation of the big toe is excellent for relieving head tension and headaches.

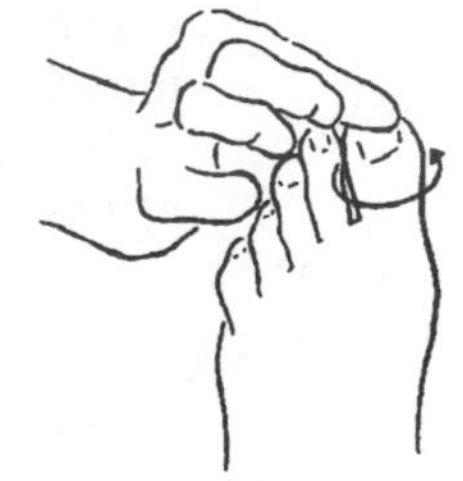

12. End by holding the whole foot again, sandwiched between your hands.

13. Repeat these strokes on the other foot.

18

Massaging the Face and Neck

In a healthy well-integrated body the head sits lightly and moves with freedom on the physical structure, allowing the face an expression of clarity, vitality and openness.... Unfortunately, life without spirit or direction..., stress and bad postural habits cause the weight of the head to fall forward, and the image and personality change. When a person is over-stressed and inactive, the weight of the head becomes a burden, putting strain on the superficial muscles of the neck.....The muscles shorten as the shoulders pull up and round, the head hangs forward, cutting off the supply of blood, nutrition and energy to the brain and causing headaches, eye strain and a general lack of spirit. The expression of the face will reflect the distress and lifelessness. The face gives an outward expression to our inner being, to the clarity of our mental activity and emotions. We have little control over the way our outer appearance maps an impression of our inner energy. It can reveal dominance with an empty, hard stare. It can shape a blank mask to hide our fear or hold a fixed and angry look to keep people at a distance. Each of these expressions reveals more than we realise about our inner state. [1]

■ The Neck

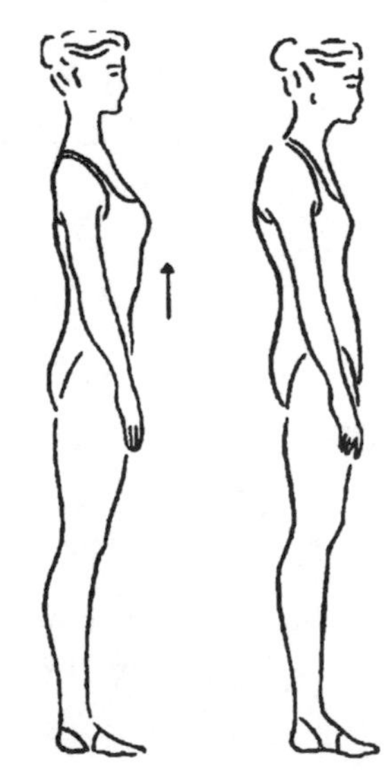

Our necks and heads are often the centre of much stress and tension. Tightness in the muscles of the neck will affect the flow of blood to the head and can cause headaches, and those 'heavy' or 'wound up' feelings. A relaxing neck massage can therefore be very releasing, stretching the spine and surrounding muscles so that the person feels 'taller' and more open.

1. Ken Eyerman (1987).

1. Although neck and face massage can be done with the person sitting up, it is more effective and relaxing if she can lie down and, if possible, close her eyes. Stand, sit or kneel comfortably at the top of her head.

2. First make some gentle contact with the person for a few seconds, so that you can focus on her and her needs. You could place your hands on either side of her head, or gently take the weight of her head with your hands, underneath the base of the skull.

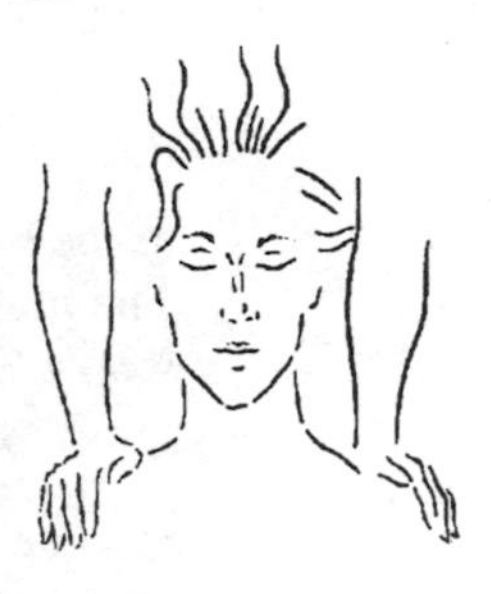

3. Having rubbed some oil onto your hands, place both hands at the base of the neck with the fingers facing inwards. Keeping your fingers on either side of the spine, draw them up under the neck all the way up to the two dents that you can feel at the top of the neck and base of the head. Do not place pressure directly onto the spine but feel your way slowly and smoothly along the muscles on either side. As you become more confident you can lift the neck slightly upwards and back to give it a gentle stretch. Do this several times. Encourage the person not to lift her head for you but to keep it relaxed and heavy.

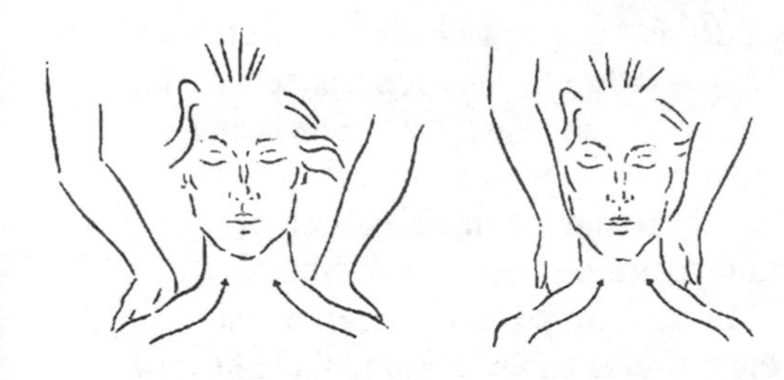

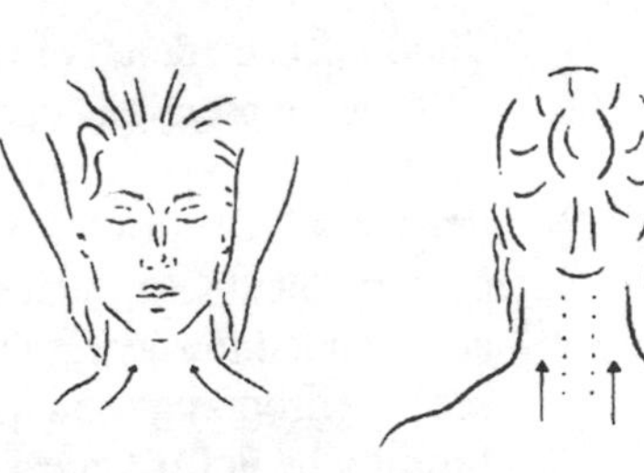

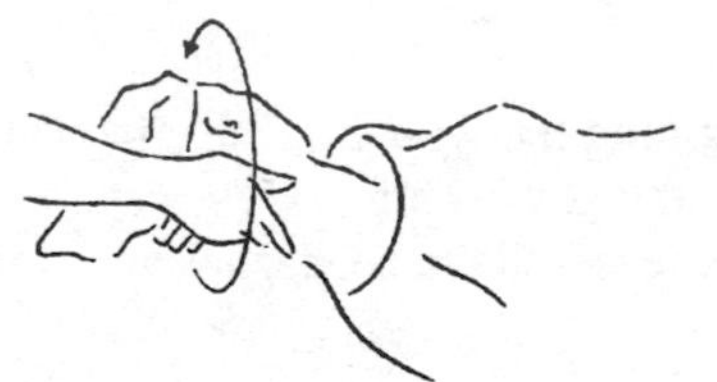

4. When your hands reach the top of the neck for the last time gently lift the head a little and turn it to the left, so that your left hand is supporting it underneath, cupping the ear.

5. Place your right hand at the top of the neck behind the ear with your fingers pointing downwards. With the bridge of your hand between the thumb and forefinger stroke down the same muscles on the right side of the cervical (neck) spine. Follow them down to the base of the neck and then on along the top of the shoulder. The muscles are often tight and may well feel lumpy. Do not worry, you will find that the bumps ease as you smooth the muscles. Repeat this several times.

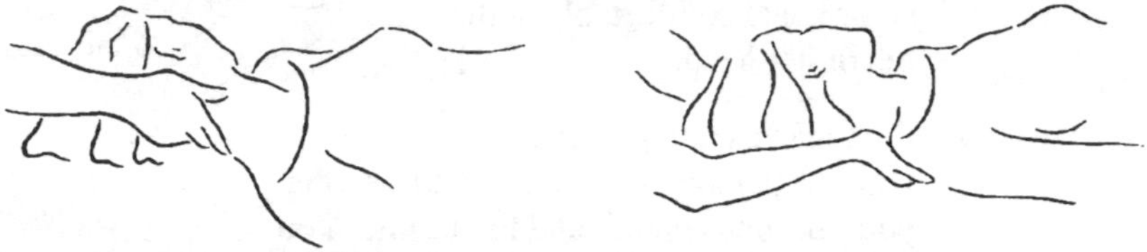

6. Holding the head again turn it now slowly to the right and repeat the previous strokes with your left hand on the left side of the back of the neck. Be careful not to press into the neck with your thumbs as the side of the neck is sensitive and contains major blood vessels.

7. Return the head to centre.

■ The Face

The face is made up of many different tiny muscles which learn to hold our expressions in certain ways. Looks of joy, surprise, shock, sadness and anger are all produced by facial muscles. Stress and tension affect muscles of the face as they do other muscle groups causing them to tighten or slacken so that the muscles become accustomed to staying in certain positions - permanent frowns, scowls, drooping mouth etc. Massage to the face, therefore, can literally be uplifting, easing the muscles and reminding them how to be relaxed and happy!

Work sensitively, but firmly, imagining that you are reshaping the face, paying particular attention to the jaw, eyebrows, eyes and temples, helping to smooth away stress, relieve headaches and clear sinuses.

1. Remain sitting or standing at the person's head and maintain even pressure. Place your hands (facing inwards) underneath the chin and draw them slowly up either side of the face to the ears. Then, starting with your thumbs together at the centre of the forehead,

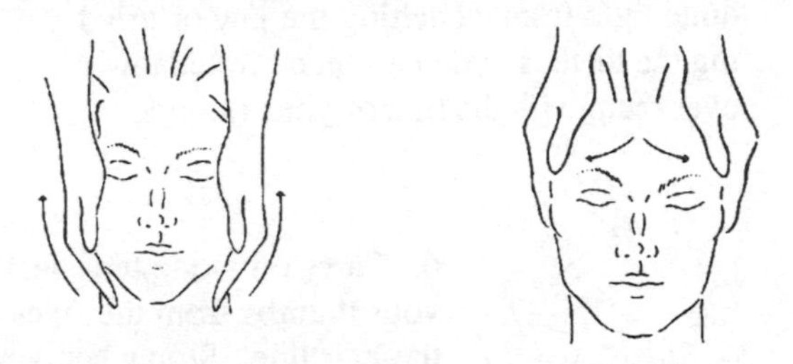

stroke both thumbs at once outwards across the forehead. Alternating these two strokes is wonderfully relaxing, and sets the pace for the rest of the massage. Repeat several times.

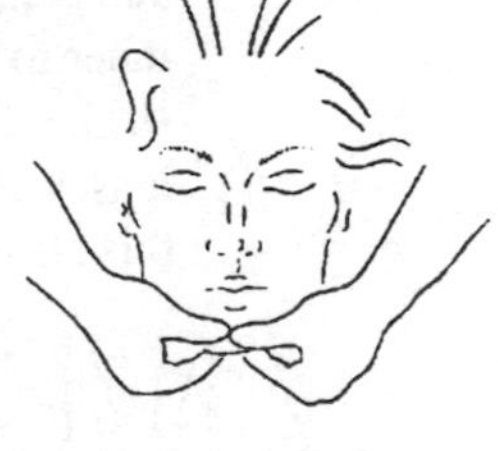

2. Now pinch lightly all around the base of the lower jaw and chin from one ear round to the other with your thumbs and fingertips.

3. In the same way as you stroked the forehead, place your thumbs together in the middle under the bottom lip. Draw them outwards pulling upwards into a smile as you reach the corners of the mouth. Encourage the person to relax her jaw by opening her mouth.

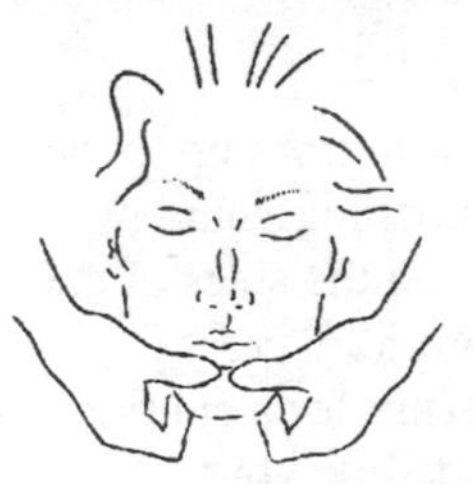

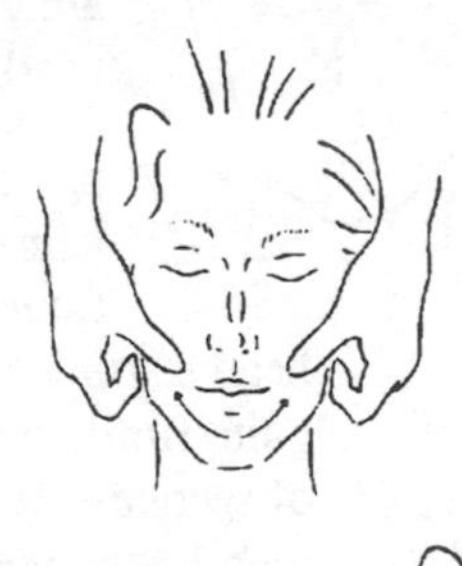

4. Do the same around the top lip underneath the nose.

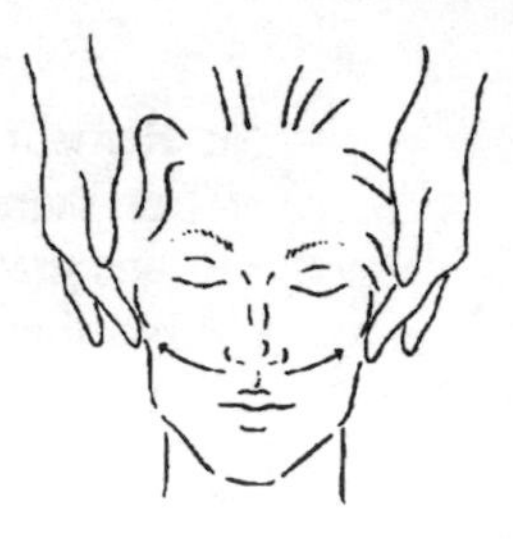

5. Beginning at the corners of the nose stroke your thumbs below the cheekbone following the line of the cheekbone to the ears. The chewing muscles there are often quite tight from clenching the jaw or grinding the teeth, so you can then circle slowly over them with the tips of your fingers.

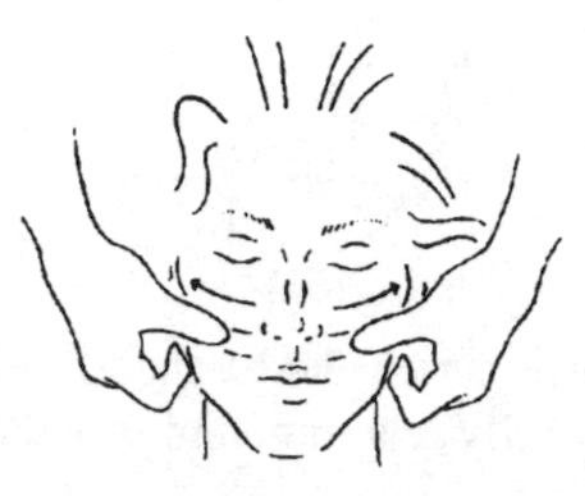

6. Carry on along the cheekbone stroking your thumbs from the sides of the nose out to the hair line. Stop when you reach the very soft delicate skin under the eyes.

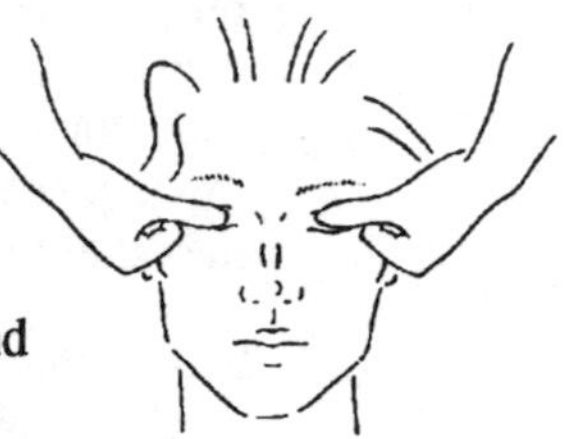

7. You can draw your thumbs lightly and gently over the eyelids from the inner to the outer corners. Avoid this stroke if the person is wearing contact lenses and be aware that some people find this stroke uncomfortable and intrusive.

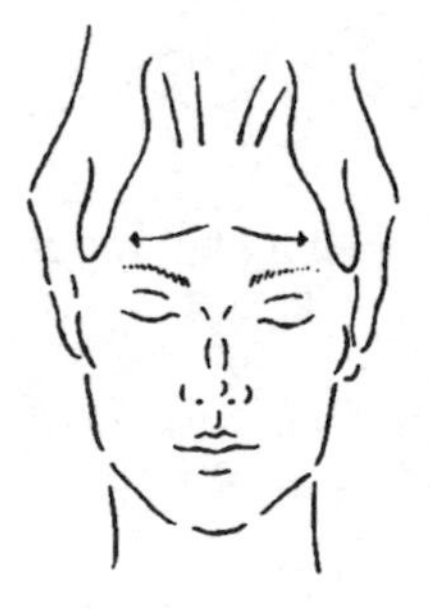

8. Move your thumbs up to the forehead and stroke outwards several times.

9. Pressure points. The following pressure points are very good for headaches, eye strain, sinuses and head colds.

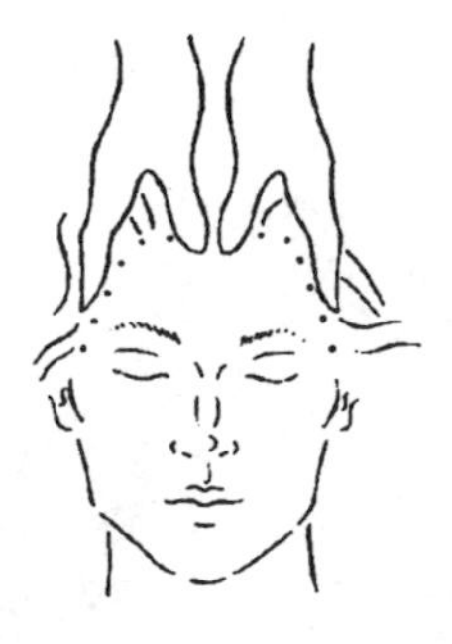

a. Move your thumbs up to the hair line and keeping your fingers gently on the sides of the head starting from the middle, press in quite firmly but not sharply for a couple of seconds. Release and slide your thumbs about 1cm apart and press again. Repeat this all around the hair line until you get down to the temples and circle them gently a couple of times.

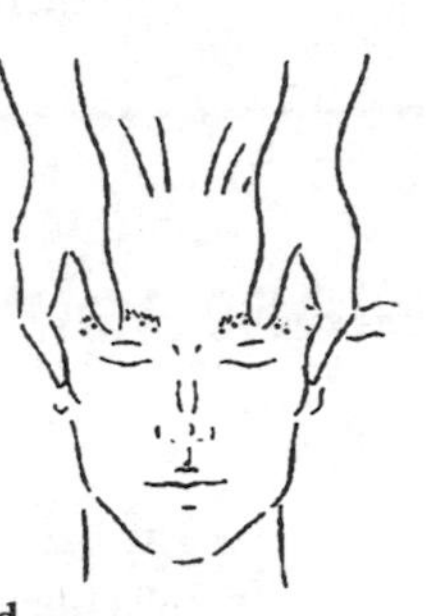

b. Still keeping your fingers on the sides of the head, place your thumbs side by side between the eyebrows. Press firmly and release. Move your thumbs down to the bony rims of the eyesockets where they connect with the nose. Press firmly for a couple of seconds and release. Now move them up along the upper half of each rim below the eyebrow hairline. Press again and repeat until you reach the temples. If the person has sinus problems these points may well be tender - the pressure can help to clear them.

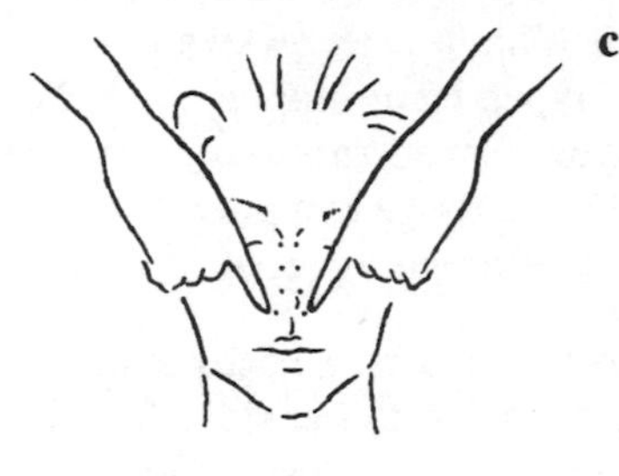

c. Now place the tips of your forefingers close beside the nose, by the corners of each eye. Press firmly and release; slide your fingers a quarter of the way down the nose and repeat. Repeat until you reach the bottom of the nose. If the person has a blocked nose or difficulty breathing through the nose these points may help to clear it.

10. End by repeating (1) several times and then gently place a cupped hand over each ear for 15-30 seconds letting the person enjoy the stillness.

19

Massaging the Back and Shoulders

The back is a really important part of the body. Down the middle runs the spine, which supplies nerves to each organ of the body. Tension in the muscles along the back and close to the spine can affect the healthy functioning of these nerves, and working on the lower back can improve a condition such as constipation. The spine also affects posture. Curvature may be aggravated by tension in the muscles surrounding the spine, holding it in an awkward position. Many postural problems can be helped by massaging the back. Most people have had a stiff neck or experienced tightness or soreness in their shoulders. Back and shoulder massage can provide immediate relief and on a regular basis can give on-going relief.

1. To massage the back effectively, the person needs to be lying down on her front with her arms down by her side. If this is not possible get her as comfortable as you can, using pillows or cushions so that as much of the back is exposed as possible.

2. By kneeling close to the side of the person you will be able to reach from the base of the spine to the neck using your body to apply pressure through your arms by moving your back and hips. In this way the massage can flow like a dance without being tiring for you.

3. Pour a small amount of oil onto your hands, *briefly* rubbing your hands together first in order to warm the oil, and then spreading your hands over the person's back to distribute the oil evenly. Begin with a long smooth stroke from the base of the back to the top of the shoulders, placing your hands on either side of the spine (never apply pressure directly onto the spine) with your fingers pointing up to the

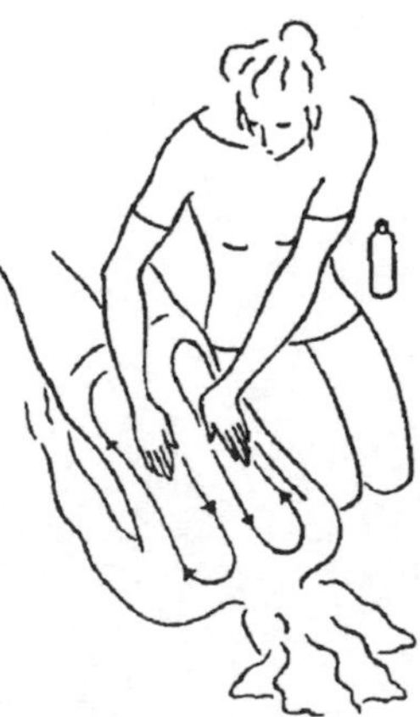

neck. Keeping your fingers together so that your hand is one continuous surface glide both your hands firmly up the entire length of the back. Try to keep your pressure even so that you apply the same amount at the top as you did at the bottom and try to keep your whole hand in contact so that you are not pushing either with your fingers or the heel of your hand. Separate your hands when you reach the shoulders and slide them between the shoulder blades and out over the top of the shoulders. Then bring the hands lightly back down to the base and start again. By using a firm stroke up the back and a lighter one down, you improve the flow of blood back to the heart. Repeat this stroke several times. It is very effective and relaxing. This stroke can also be used on the legs and arms, always making a firm stroke towards the heart and a light one on the return journey.

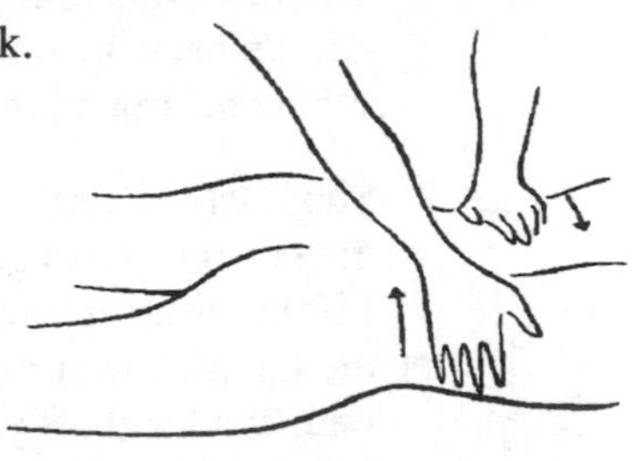

4. Now move down to the lower back. Place your left hand on the person's nearest side with your fingers pointing across the back, and place your right hand on the far side with your fingers pointing down. Keeping your pressure even with both hands, push your left hand firmly forward over the back to the other side and at the same time pull your right hand back towards you. Without stopping, change direction, bringing the hands back to the original position. Repeat this, working up the lower back, keeping the wringing movement flowing and the pressure even. By moving your body at the hips it is possible to create a smooth rhythm. Most people find this stroke very soothing. Return lightly with a single stroke.

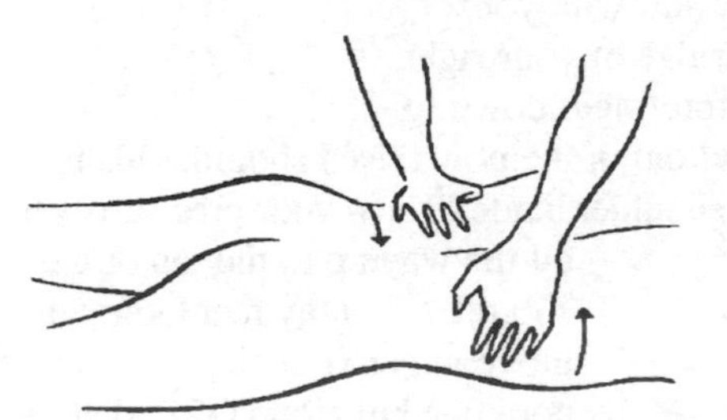

5. The next stroke is deeper and should be introduced gradually if you want to release hidden tension in deeper tissues. Begin working on the muscles on either side of the spine. Kneeling on one side by the centre of the person's back, place the heel of your

hand next to the opposite side of the spine in the space between the muscles and the spine, with your fingers pointing down towards the far side. Push into and over the muscle with the heel of your right hand continuing out over the right side. Work up the right side of the spine, lifting your hand off to repeat the stroke, being careful not to place pressure directly on the spine. Use your other hand as a brace a bit further up the back or alternate the movement with both hands. Repeat on the other side.

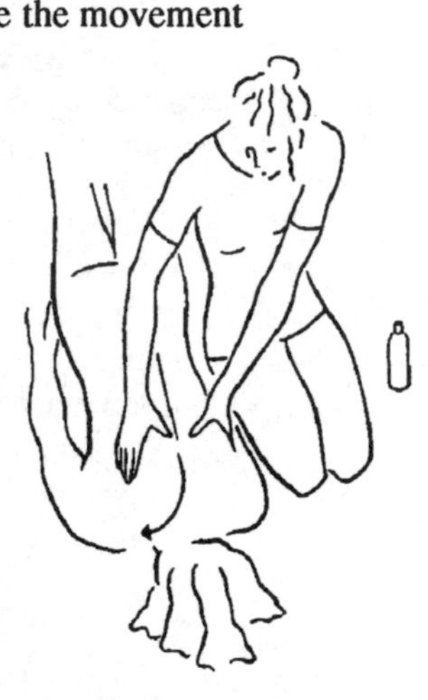

6. To relieve tension along the upper part of the spine, run your thumbs from the middle back up along the edge of the spine and around the shoulder.

7. Shoulders. Kneel on one side and turn the person's head gently away from you. Lift her nearest forearm backwards onto the middle lower back and support it with one hand. If you are working on the left shoulder, support her arm with your left hand and place the bridge of your right hand (the line along the forefinger down to the thumb) against the bottom of the now raised shoulder blade. Stroke up and round the shoulder blade. Keep your pressure even all the way up to the top of the shoulder. It may feel lumpy or move under your fingers. This is not bone but a good sign that the tense muscles are relaxing and 'letting go'. Repeat this several times. Replace the arm then move round to the other side and repeat the movement on the other shoulder, after turning the person's head.

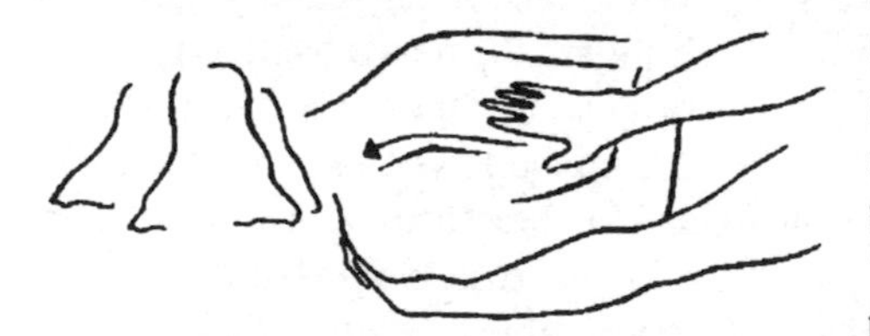

8. Cupping. This movement is invigorating. Avoid cupping if the person is nervous, upset or if your aim is to relax her. As it is very stimulating it is good for people who have difficulty

coughing up phlegm or who have a lot of tension in their back. Cup your hands, arching them with your fingers together so that there is a hollow in the palms of your hands. Keeping your wrists loose, bounce your hands alternately and fairly rapidly up and down over the fleshy area of the back and up over the shoulders. This stroke helps to loosen and stimulate the underlying tissues improving the circulation and loosening catarrh.

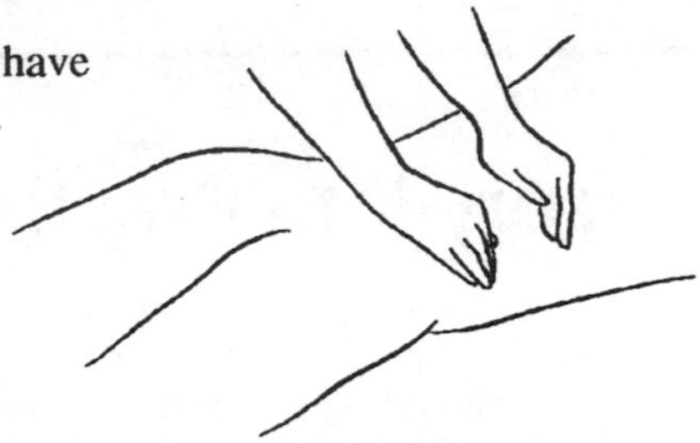

9. Whether or not cupping is appropriate, use slow calming strokes (as in 3 above) to finish the massage.

20

Theory Into Practice

The following examples illustrate the authors' experiences of using aromatherapy and massage with people who have learning difficulties. They have been supplemented by the experiences of nurses, teachers, support staff, day centre officers, occupational therapists and physiotherapists in a range of settings; home, community, day centres and hospitals, with adults and children. Some of the people have a formal qualification in aromatherapy and massage; many have attended a one day workshop.

All the names have been changed and a little editing has been undertaken in order that the examples follow a similar style. The examples have not been arranged into any categories as this would seem to be somewhat artificial. Of course it could be argued that the attention of another person, the environment and other circumstances have played a significant role. That is not disputed. It is hoped that these examples of what has happened when massage, with and without essential oils, has been used in the lives of people with learning difficulties, may encourage others to seek the same benefits for the people they support.

■ Joanne

Joanne attends the 'special needs unit' at her local adult training centre where the physiotherapist works with her on a regular basis. She has no communication other than body language and tends to withdraw into a corner and cover herself with blankets and cushions. She dislikes being in a group and spends much of her time picking up small pieces of paper and fabric which she holds in her fist, then pulls her hands up into her jumper sleeves.

If this behaviour is disturbed, Joanne will scream and injure herself with her nails. She prefers to be by herself and avoids eye contact. Her frequent outbursts of temper seem to be related either to headaches or pre-menstrual tension. The physiotherapist used massage to try to help Joanne to accept touch without self injury, and to encourage her to use her hands to explore the environment and extend her horizons through touch. To do this she took Joanne daily to a secure and restful setting. A small room next to the 'special needs unit' was regularly used for relaxation and sensory awareness. The physiotherapist attempted to massage Joanne's hands, feet, neck and face using relaxing essential oils. In the long term she hoped to help Joanne achieve a degree of relaxation which was not dependent on the setting and to encourage her to associate the smell of essential oils with pleasure and relaxation.

Working with the staff of the adult training centre, Joanne's behaviour was monitored, and this showed a definite increase in outbursts of temper immediately prior to menstruation. Rose oil diluted in a carrier oil was therefore used prior to menstruation with good effect. Eventually all that was necessary was for the day centre officer to apply the oil to Joanne's hands as soon as she arrived at the 'special needs unit' and this enabled her to relax. Joanne began to sit for periods of the day without covering herself with blankets and appeared to be generally happier. She also began to sit and use one hand for a simple constructive activity rather than just picking up fluff and pieces of paper.

■ Tanya

Tanya has dual sensory impairment and is unsteady on her feet. She hangs her head and spends most of the time curled up. She becomes very frustrated when she can't walk as easily as she would like and, when tense, punches her head. The massage therapist was asked into her flat by her support workers, who felt that massage might relax her, improve her responsiveness and possibly help her mobility. The massage therapist started by gently massaging her feet and legs. On the first occasion she kicked out when her toes were touched, but the next time she quickly relaxed and seemed to sense that it was doing her some good. When the massage therapist took her hands away she would reach out for them and put them back on her legs. The massage therapist taught the support staff how to do hand, foot and face massage and they now regularly massage her. She loves and thrives on the contact and will settle immediately if massaged when distressed. She is now walking independently using a trail rail around her flat and parts of the residential site.

■ Simon

Simon is 18 months old. He has spasticity in each limb and cries continuously unless he is sitting on his mother's lap. The nurse who worked with him aimed to help him to improve his hand co-ordination, as Simon was unable to reach and grasp a rattle without going into contraction.

In the first session, whilst Simon sat on his mother's lap, the nurse massaged his hands and arms. He responded by staring intently at his hands and then at the nurse. Almost immediately he tried to stroke her hands in imitation. After ten minutes his mother had to answer the phone and placed Simon on the carpet. Although the nurse had been visiting Simon and his mother for five months it was the first time that he did not become distressed. The nurse continued to massage his back and stomach. Simon enjoyed ten minutes of massage whilst his mother was on the telephone. It was also interesting that he opened his hand to grasp a rattle and returned it with a deliberate and easy motion. This skill was only evident after a hand massage with relaxing essential oil of lavender with black pepper. Usually Simon woke three to four times every night but after a hand massage he would sleep through the night. His mother now massages him twice a week with similar good results.

■ Christine

Christine is an 8 year old girl who has profound learning difficulties and has spasticity in her legs and arms. She has no vision and cannot control her head. She does not enjoy good health and is frequently absent from school as she has regular chest infections and her skin breaks down easily. She is also prone to eye infections.

At school she is stimulated through a sensory approach to learning. She appears to enjoy singing; when she is sung to she makes happy sing-song noises in response. Christine totally relaxes in the hydrotherapy pool. The aims of including aromatherapy in this sensory approach were to:

> *Promote better health, to keep her chest clear and reduce the incidence of eye and ear infections.*
>
> *To offer Christine more opportunities for close non-verbal communication*
>
> *To encourage responses and eventual anticipation of the activity.*

During aromatherapy sessions Christine was undressed, laid on her stomach on a bed and covered with warm towels. A relaxing combination of lavender and chamomile essential oils, also known for their antiseptic qualities, were used, to which a few drops of eucalyptus were added to reduce infection. When Christine was offered the oil mixture to smell she cooed and gurgled and her nostrils flared. Her back was then massaged for 20 minutes by the end of which Christine had often fallen asleep. During sessions when she did not fall asleep, Christine responded with increased vocalisation to having her legs and feet massaged and moved her whole body in apparent pleasure and enjoyment.

Later, massage was introducсd to her face and chest and eventually covered the whole of her body. A more invigorating essential oil was substituted for lavender to help Christine to stay awake during the whole massage. Soon Christine began to show anticipation of a pleasurable aromatherapy session by flaring her nostrils, cooing and gurgling at the beginning of the session.

■ Mohammed

Mohammed is a 26 year old man who is described as having challenging behaviour and severe learning difficulties. When Mohammed becomes upset he will often spit, pinch and bite the staff who work with him on the wards of the hospital where he lives. In the past it has been assumed that he enjoys solitude and his own company because he will often take himself off and sit alone.

The occupational therapist (O.T.) treated the spasticity in his muscles by going through passive exercises with Mohammed which he tolerated. When the O.T. became interested in aromatherapy she began to introduce hand massage when she saw him twice a week. Mohammed initially just tolerated his hands being touched in the same way that he appeared to tolerate passive movements, although he would occasionally withdraw his hands. Gradually the O.T. began to massage his feet as well as his hands. He appeared to enjoy these sessions and offered his hands to be massaged. The O.T. used a combination of the relaxing essential oils of lavender and marjoram and also included a few drops of eucalyptus as Mohammed suffers from sinus problems.

On one occasion when Mohammed appeared to be agitated and had scratched a member of staff and spat at another person, the O.T. decided to continue the massage session and began by putting the massage oil close to Mohammed's nose for him to smell. The O.T. massaged his feet and then Mohammed offered his hands to be massaged after which he remained quiet and relaxed for twenty minutes. As Mohammed appeared to find this combination of essential oils and massage relaxing, it was hoped the oils could begin to be used in the bath, as he becomes agitated and distressed when he takes a bath.

■ Matthew

Matthew is a 29 year old man who attends a 'multisensory room' with an O.T. once a week to help him to relax. Although registered blind with severe learning difficulties, Matthew has some vision. He is easily startled and becomes quickly distressed when approached or touched. When distressed Matthew chews his clothes. When Matthew first began to use the multisensory room with the O.T. he would curl up with his face downwards and reject any interaction. After a number of weeks he was able to lie on the matting and relax, lying down for up to 40 minutes. The O.T. massaged his hands and feet using relaxing essential oils, and noticed a gradual increase in his tolerance to touch and acceptance of the presence of others. He is not startled as easily and the incidence of chewing his clothes has decreased during the sessions.

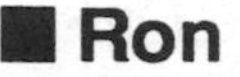

Ron

Ron is a young man with learning difficulties who has spent the majority of his life in a hospital. His closest friend is Peter who lives in the same house on the hospital grounds. Together they attend a weekly yoga and relaxation class which uses massage to promote relaxation. Ron has quite severe physical disabilities which means that he moves in a wheelchair with little movement in his hands and legs. He also has a large amount of scar tissue from burns on his feet. Relaxation for both these young men seemed initially problematic. It was difficult to explain what was meant by relaxation as both had quite severe communication difficulties.

Many strategies were tried, for example, a different and slower music tape from that used for the yoga postures was used. The staff modelled the behaviour, demonstrating relaxing on pillows, mats and bean bags. The two men often appeared to sabotage the efforts for peace and relaxation when one of them would burst out laughing - which inevitably set others off giggling. Through trial and error the relaxation sessions were extended from 30 seconds to a regular 5 to 6 minutes. It was important to time the sessions to give a sense of achievement as it took many months to achieve 5 minutes of relaxation regularly.

The successful strategies were with music which clearly promoted a change of mood. On a couple of occasions a different relaxation tape was used but Ron clearly protested by continually lifting his head and scowling. Massage using lavender oil was very successful. It took some time to find the areas which gave the most relaxed response. For Ron this was his feet. He could be restless when unsettled but always responded well to foot massage. Peter achieved this through back massage. The relaxation sessions were carried out by a nurse and Peter's key worker. The sessions strengthened their friendship with each other and all four found the weekly period of relaxation to be mutually beneficial.

Jenny

Jenny is a 55 year old woman who has lived in hospital since she was 15 years old. Her father died fourteen years ago and her mother before that. Jenny communicates easily but often prefers to sit alone, withdrawing and isolating herself from other people. She appears to be tense and rigid, holding her arms tightly to her body. In the past she enjoyed singing and dancing to music, when she would smile, laugh and enjoy people's company, but recently she has not wanted to join in. There is a relaxation group on the ward run by the O.T.. Jenny was asked if she would like to attend to encourage her to be with other people, offering her an opportunity to express her emotions and to allow her to relax.

The group began with an opportunity to smell different essential oils. People in the group felt the different textures of talc, oil and lotion rubbed on the back of their hands so that each member could choose which she wanted for the massage. Initially Jenny chose talc to be massaged into her hand. For a few seconds Jenny allowed the back of her left hand to be rubbed with talc and then she withdrew her hand. Over the next two sessions the time increased and her right hand was also massaged for a couple of minutes. As her tolerance increased she chose oil as the medium and allowed her key worker to give her a ten minute massage on each hand. She told the key worker that she now enjoyed the massage and sang quietly to herself as she left the session. Jenny now receives and enjoys regular hand massage, and her relationship with her key worker continues to develop as Jenny begins to open up more about herself.

■ Jill

Jill is a 48 year old woman who has severe learning difficulties and multiple disabilities. She cannot communicate verbally and is dependent on others to fulfil her needs. She uses a wheelchair and she does not have much control over her environment. As a result she has become rather isolated and spends most of her day on the ward sucking her fingers in front of the television. Jill has been receiving regular aromatherapy and massage for about a year and there has been a noticeable change in her motivation and interaction with others.

She now actively seeks attention and physical contact by vocalising loudly and stretching out her arm to people. It appears that the one-to-one attention given when receiving a massage has acted as a catalyst towards greater motivation and interaction with other people. She appears more aware of things around her and is now making simple choices about drinks and food and is more inclined to try different activities than she was previously.

Sabi

Sabi has lived for most of her life in a long stay hospital for people who have learning difficulties. She has a warm, enthusiastic personality and a mild learning difficulty. Sabi currently lives in a small home near the hospital and is preparing for a move to a new home in the community. She was very enthusiastic about having aromatherapy and keen to try massage on different parts of her body. She particularly enjoys a back massage, usually using lavender and chamomile and has noted that the tension held in her neck and shoulders is decreasing. Her skin is very dry, so a carrier oil containing essential oils which are also good for dry skin was applied to her legs lightly as she has varicose veins. A similar bath oil was made up which Sabi uses regularly with the result that her legs no longer itch and there is no dry skin as before.

Phil

Phil has profound learning difficulties and severe physical disabilities caused by meningitis. He is 7 years old and suffers from chronic constipation. His whole body is very stiff. Phil communicates by making lip smacking movements when he wants a drink, or in response to a pleasant smell, and his eyes move from side to side when someone calls his name. Aromatherapy was introduced to his curriculum at school to improve his health, in particular his circulation, to lessen constipation and improve a chest condition. It was also used to decrease stiffness, working in conjunction with the physiotherapist and to increase Phil's tolerance of being handled.

At each aromatherapy session Phil was undressed, laid on a sheepskin and covered with warm towels. A mixture of lavender, eucalyptus and marjoram was chosen to treat his physical complaints. Phil was offered the blended oils to smell and then his back was gently massaged for fifteen minutes. After this the physiotherapist began her session of stretching exercises. She noted a great change in stiffness stating that Phil was much more relaxed.

■ Peter

Peter is 26 and has severe learning difficulties, spastic quadriplegia and impaired vision. He lived with his family until he was 8 years old, when he went to a large institution until he was 24. He then moved into a small group home and now attends a day unit for people with learning difficulties. Peter spends most of his day in a chair or lying on a mat. At times, when distressed, he will bite himself or try to throw himself across the floor. In order to bring a wide range of appropriate experiences and activities into Peter's life, foot massage was introduced. Relaxing oils of lavender, geranium and marjoram were used. Peter is generally resistant to touch which makes many tasks difficult or unpleasant for him.

By trying to introduce touch as a positive experience it was hoped that his distress would decrease and Peter would begin to enjoy being touched. Initially Peter resisted all attempts at being touched, moving his feet away. After a couple of sessions he allowed his feet to be massaged for a few seconds, tolerating the touch. Now, he allows his feet to be massaged and consistently smiles during the session. He will indicate the end of the session by pushing hands away. Peter does not have natural bowel movements and stomach massage with appropriate essential oils to help regulate his movements is being introduced. Peter will now lie happily on a mat and enjoys his stomach being massaged.

■ Susan

Susan lives with her parents and attends the local adult training centre on a regular basis. At home she has a very erratic sleep pattern and her parents were distressed by Susan's aggression to other people, which often took the form of hitting passers-by with a closed fist. She appeared to be generally unco-operative at the training centre and had outbursts of temper in public. Working with the day centre officers, the physiotherapist monitored Susan's behaviour and found that there was a definite link between aggressive behaviour and premenstrual tension. The physiotherapist aimed to use massage to help Susan relax and enjoy a regular sleep pattern, and to reduce aggression by establishing 'touch' without eliciting fear. It was hoped that this would also help Susan to participate in small group activities.

To do this, the physiotherapist had a regular 20 minute session with Susan in a quiet room where she massaged her with essential oils. It was hoped to create an association between the smell of the oil and a feeling of well-being. The physiotherapist also involved Susan's mother in the programme, and she used lavender in the bath to help Susan to relax. Rose oil diluted in a carrier oil was used prior to menstruation. The quiet room was used for these sessions for two weeks. Very quickly the use of the quiet room was unnecessary. After the second session of massage, Susan slept through the night.

A few drops of lavender oil was used to fragrance the room where Susan spent the day at the training centre. The staff, physiotherapist and Susan's mother agree that, through the use of essential oils, very obvious signs of relaxation have been seen in Susan and her sleep pattern has improved. Staff changes and shortages mean that encouraging Susan to participate in small groups has temporarily broken down. However the improvements at home continue.

■ Home Visit

On a home visit to a mother who has a 12 year old boy with learning difficulties, a nurse found her in an extremely stressed and anxious condition. Her son had begun to hit out at family members. A joint visit with the psychologist accompanying the nurse was made; however the boy's mother was in no state to talk calmly about the situation. The nurse suggested a hand massage using lavender and chamomile to help her relax. She accepted in desperation although she was cynical of any positive result. After 5 minutes she visibly relaxed, her speech slowed, becoming more coherent, and she began to think positively about strategies of coping.

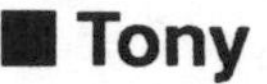

Tony

Tony has severe learning difficulties. He uses a wheelchair and has spastic tone and stiffness in his arms and legs. Tony is also prone to constipation which causes him much discomfort. The O.T.'s initial contact with Tony was to do passive exercises to decrease the spastic tone in his limbs and to improve his posture generally which, it is hoped, will decrease the risk of further deformity and associated respiratory difficulties.

As aromatherapy was introduced the O.T. began by doing hand massage. Tony's hands were very contracted, but after fifteen minutes of massage they were able to open up more than usual. Tony also appeared to be very relaxed. Foot massage was also introduced and similarly, Tony appeared to be relaxed and found it enjoyable. The essential oils used were lavender, marjoram and chamomile to relax the spasticity in Tony's muscles and help treat his constipation. As the oils are antiseptic they were excellent for Tony's hands which, because they were constantly clenched due to spasticity, became sweaty, hot and prone to sores. Tony receives aromatherapy treatments of hand and foot massage once a week. His hands are more relaxed and his constipation has improved.

■ Joe

Joe is 24 and has spastic tone in his legs and arms. He has regular sessions with an O.T. who uses a multisensory room to help Joe relax. The room is small and has varied lighting effects, music and tactile stimuli. The O.T. uses massage with relaxing essential oils for Joe and also burns relaxing oils. Joe has some voluntary movement in his left arm and hand and often pinches and hits himself with it.

During the weekly massage session in the multisensory room, Joe sits supported by pillows and the O.T. massages his hands, arms, neck and scalp. Joe also listens to relaxing music and makes giggling vocalisations which he usually does when he is happy. If agitated on arrival he quickly appears to relax. As well as being able to enjoy relaxation, the incidence of self injurious behaviour has significantly decreased both at home and during the sessions.

■ A Final Word

A final word from a day centre officer in London who has been using aromatherapy there for over three years:

> Many of the people with learning difficulties develop simple massage techniques so they can massage others. Parents and carers have used the oils within their homes and reported positive results with aromatherapy in reducing stress... There is very little scepticism among those who have had the opportunity of observing the reactions of people who have gone into an aromatherapy session in a very challenging frame of mind and have emerged relaxed and calm.

Glossary of Terms

Carrier Oil

A greasy, unperfumed vegetable oil which nourishes the skin and can have slight therapeutic properties of its own. It is used to give the necessary lubrication in a massage oil.

Carrier Lotion

A non-greasy, unperfumed simple oil and water emulsion used to blend with essential oils for application to the body. Also helps to improve skin texture.

Complementary Medicine

This covers an almost endless range of techniques and therapies which, by treating causes rather than symptoms, affect the whole person's mind, body and spirit, stimulating an intrinsic ability to self-heal.

Essential Oil

A fragrant essence which is extracted from an aromatic plant by steam distillation or expression (citrus oils). Each oil has its own therapeutic properties.

Interactive Massage

The emphasis for this type of massage is not on providing a passive, relaxing experience, but on using massage as an opportunity to share and communicate. This involves encouraging the person to imitate massage movements on your hand and to lead the session by showing you where to massage. The interactive sequence provides a guide to the stages that a person may go through in order to do this.

Massage Oil

A carrier oil to which essential oils have been added.

Multisensory Massage

The use of different textures or massage tools and essential oils to provide a sensory stimulation for people who have severe or profound learning difficulties. This could be a passive or interactive experience, depending on the person's needs.

Perfume Oil

This is usually a synthetic perfume in an oil base which can be used either as a perfume or in a burner. It does not have any therapeutic qualities.

Reflexology

This therapy is based on the principle that all organs and parts of the body are mirrored in the feet. By applying pressure to the corresponding area, or reflex point, it is possible to improve a person's health.

Shiatsu

A Japanese therapy which involves applying finger pressure to acupuncture points along energy channels throughout the body, called meridians, to promote a balance of energy and good health.

Bibliography

Ayres, J. (1972) Sensory Integration and Learning Disorders. *Western Psychological Services, California.*

Bardeau, F. (1976) La Medicine Aromatique. *Robert Lafont.*

Bernadet, M. La Phyto-aromatherapie Pratique. *Dangles.*

Bijou, S.W. (1966) A Functional Analysis of Retarded Development. In: International Review of Research in Mental Retardation, M.R. Ellis (Ed), pp 62-71. *Academic Press, New York.*

Birchall, A. (1990) A Whiff of Happiness. *New Scientist, 25th August 1990.*

Brandon, D. and Brandon, A. (1986) Putting People First; A Handbook on the Practical Application of Ordinary Living Principles. *Good Impressions Publishing Ltd., London.*

Brandon, D. (1989) How Gentle Teaching Can Liberate Us All. *Community Living, April 1990.*

Brandon, D. (1989) Gentle Teaching. *Nursing Times, Vol. 86 No. 2.*

Bronfenbrenner, V. (1974) as cited in McInnes, J and Treffry, J. (1982) Deaf-Blind Infants and Children - A Developmental Guide. *Open University Press, Milton Keynes.*

Coupe, J. et al (1985) The Affective Communication Assessment. *Special Education, Manchester.*

Davison, K. (1990) Reaching Out to Anorexic Patients. *Therapy Weekly, November 1st 1990.*

Downing, G. (1972) The Massage Book. *Arkana.*

Durrafourd, P. (1982) En Forme Tous Les Jours. *Cevic.*

Eyerman, K. (1987) Massage. *Sidgwick and Jackson.*

Farrow, J. (1990) Massage Therapy and Nursing Care. *Nursing Standard, Volume 4/17.*

Favell, J.E., McGimsey, J.F. and Schell, R.M. (1982) Treatment of Self Injury by providing Alternative Sensory Activity. *Analysis and Intervention on Developmental Disabilities. Vol. 2, 83-104.*

Harlow, H.F. (1965) cited in Montague, A. (1986) Touching - The Human Significance of the Skin. *Harper and Row, New York.*

Harrison, J.S. (1984) An Evaluation of Different Approaches to the Understanding and Treatment of Self Injury with Particular Reference to People who are Mentally Handicapped. *Unpublished dissertation.*

Hogg, J., Sebba, J. and Lambe, L. (1990) Profound Retardation and Multiple Impairment. Vol. 3, Medical and Physical Care and Management. *Chapman and Hall, London.*

Holmes, P. (1986) Fringe Benefits. *Nursing Times. Vol. 28, 20-22.*

Hooper, A. (1988) Massage and Loving. *Unwin Hyman Ltd., London.*

Jones, R. (1990) Gentle Teaching - Behaviourism at its Best. *Community Living, January 1990.*

Kings Fund Centre (1989) Ties and Connections - an Ordinary Community Life for People with Learning Difficulties. *Kings Fund, London.*

Kirsta, A. (1986) The Book of Stress Survival. *Guild Publishing, London.*

Knickerbocker, B.M. (1980) A Holistic Approach to the Treatment of Learning Disorders. *New York.*

Lake, M. (1990) Scents amd Sensuality. *John Murray, London.*

Lidell, L. (1984) The Book of Massage. *Gaia Books, London.*

Longhorn, F. (1988) A Sensory Curriculum for Very Special People. *Souvenir Press, London.*

Lautie, R. and Passebecq, A. Aromatherapy. *Out of print.*

Maybey, R. The Complete New Herbal. *Elm Tree Books.*

McGee, J. et al (1987) Gentle Teaching - A Non-Aversive Approach to Helping Persons with Mental Retardation. *Human Sciences Press.*

McInnes, J. and Treffry, J. (1982) Deaf-Blind Infants and Children - A Developmental Guide. *Open University Press, Milton Keynes.*

McCray, G. (1978) cited in Montague, A. (1986) Touching - The Human Significance of the Skin. *Harper and Row, New York.*

McPhail, C. and Chamore, A. (1989) Relaxation Reduces Disruption in Mentally Handicapped Adults. *Journal of Mental Deficiency Research, 33, 399-406.*

Montague, A. (1986) Touching - The Human Significance of the Skin. *Harper and Row, New York.*

O'Brien, J. (1986) A Comprehensive Guide to the Activities Catalogue: An Alternative Curriculum for Youths and Adults with Severe Learning Difficulties. In: Bellamy, J.T. and Wilcox, B. (Eds). Baltimore, Maryland. *Paul H. Brooks (Publisher).*

Oliver, L. (1987) Meditation and the Creative Imperative. *Dryad Press.*

Ouvry, C. (1987) Educating Children with Profound Handicaps. *BIMH Publications, Kidderminster.*

Passant, H. (1990) Complementary Therapies - A Holistic Approach on the Ward. *Nursing Times, Vol. 86, No. 4.*

Peck, C. (1977) Desensitisation for the Treatment of Fear in the High Level Adult Retardate. *Behaviour, Research and Therapy, 15.*

Prescot, J. (1963) cited in Montague, A. (1986) Touching - The Human Significance of the Skin. *Harper and Row, New York.*

Price, S. (1983) Practical Aromatherapy. *Harper and Collins Group, London*

Price, S. (1991) Aromatherapy and Common Ailments. *Gaia Books, London.*

Provence, S. and Lipton, R.C. (1962) cited in Montague, A. (1986) Touching - The Human Significance of the Skin. *Harper and Row, New York.*

Rouviere, A. and Meyer, M.C. (1983) Les Huiles Essentielles. *M. A. Editions.*

Rovesti, P. (1971) cited in Tisserand, R. (1988) Aromatherapy for Everyone. *Penguin Books, London.*

Sanderson, H.L. and Gitsham, N. (1990) A Holistic Sensory Approach - A Guide to Sensory Stimulation for People Who Have Learning Disabilities. *Oxford Health Authority.*

Sanderson Turnbull, J. (1990) Aromatherapy and its Implications for Profoundly Handicapped Children. *Unpublished dissertation.*

Sandman, C.A. et al (1983) Naloxone Attenuates Self-Abusive Behaviour in Developmentally Disabled Clients. *Applied Research in Mental Retardation. 4.1.*

Shevrin, A. and Toussieng, P.W. (1965) cited in Montague, A. Touching - The Human Significance of the Skin. *Harper and Row, New York.*

Sims, S. Slow Stroke Massage for Cancer Patients. *Nursing Times. Vol. 82, 47-50.*

Smith, M. (1990) Healing Through Touch. *Nursing Times Vol. 86, No. 4.*

Spitz, R. (1946) cited in Montague, A. (1986) Touching - The Human Significance of the Skin. *Harper and Row, New York.*

Steen, P. and Zuriff, G. (1977) The Use of Relaxation in the Treatment of Self Injurious Behaviour. *Journal of Behaviour Therapy and Experimental Psychiatry. 8, 447-448.*

Thomas, M. (1989) Fancy Footwork. *Nursing Times. Vol. 85, No. 41.*

Tisserand, R. (1988) Aromatherapy for Everyone. *Penguin Books, London.*

Turton, P. (1989) Therapeutic Touch: Its Place in Nursing Care. In: Pritchard, A.P. (Ed.) Cancer Nursing - A Revolution in Care: Proceedings of the Fifth International Conference on Cancer Nursing. *MacMillan, London.*

Valnet, J. (1980) The Practice Of Aromatherapy. *C.W. Daniel Co. Ltd.*

Van Toller, S and Dodd, G. (1988) Perfumery: The Psychology and Biology of Fragrance. *Chapman and Hall, London.*

Wells, K., Turner, S., Bellack, A. and Hersen, M. (1978) Effects of Cue-Controlled Relaxation and Psychomotor Seizures: and Experimental Analysis. *Behaviour Research and Therapy. 16, 51-53.*

Zigler, E. (1966) Research on Personality Structure in the Retardate. In: International Review of Research in Mental Retardation. Ellis, M. (Ed.) pp 194-199. *Academic Press, New York.*

Further Reading

Brandon, D. and Brandon, A. (1986) Putting People First; A Handbook on the Practical Application of Ordinary Living Principles. *Good Impressions Publishing Ltd., London.*

Davis, P. (1988) Aromatherapy, An A-Z. *C.W. Daniel Co. Ltd.*

Kings Fund Centre (1989) Ties and Connections - an Ordinary Community Life for People with Learning Difficulties. *Kings Fund, London.*

Lidell, L. (1984) The Book of Massage. *Gaia Books, London.*

McInnes, J. and Treffry, J. (1982) Deaf-Blind Infants and Children - A Developmental Guide. *Open University Press, Milton Keynes.*

Montagu, A. (1986) Touching - The Human Significance of the Skin. *Harper and Row, New York.*

Price, S. (1983) Practical Aromatherapy. *Harper and Collins Group, London.*

Price, S. (1991) Aromatherapy and Common Ailments. *Gaia Books, London.*

Tisserand, R. (1989) The Art of Aromatherapy. *C.W. Daniel Co.*

Valnet, J. (1980) The Practice Of Aromatherapy. *C.W. Daniel Co.*

Further Information

This book is designed to accompany a one-day course and one-day follow up entitled "Aromatherapy and Massage for People with Learning Difficulties". These courses are particularly for parents and support workers who want to start using aromatherapy with people with learning difficulties. They are run regularly at four venues around the country by Helen Sanderson, Jane Harrison, Julie Lunt and Judy Ruddle who together form Hands on Training. As well as covering some of the factual information presented in the book, participants will also learn how to blend their own oils and learn the basic movements of massage described in the book. Details of these two days can be obtained from Hands on Training at the address on the next page. The courses can also be arranged at your own venue. For further details contact Helen Sanderson at the address overleaf.

Hands on Training also run a one-day course for experienced aromatherapists or massage therapists who wish to offer massage to people with learning difficulties. For further information contact Shirley Price Aromatherapy Ltd.

From 1994 Hands on Training will be joining with Advocacy in Action, a group of people with learning difficulties and their support workers, to co-run a workshop looking at issues around touch.

Shirley Price runs a number of courses on aromatherapy, including a Diploma Course for people who wish to become qualified aromatherapists. Shirley can also provide a list of all qualified aromatherapists practising in your area. She runs a mail order service supplying quality aromatherapy products. For product details and course information contact Shirley Price Aromatherapy Ltd. at the address given on the next page.

For details of a Diploma Course in Therapeutic Massage held in London and Glasgow contact The College of Holistic Medicine at the address given on the next page. The College can also provide a list of qualified therapists working in your area.

For further copies of the book contact Jane Harrison at Hands on Publishing or Shirley Price Aromatherapy Ltd.

Shirley Price Aromatherapy Ltd.
Essentia House
Upper Bond Street
Hinckley
Leicestershire LE10 1RS

Jane Harrison
Hands On Publishing
62 Sir Johns Road
Selly Park
Birmingham B29 7ER

The College of Holistic Medicine
4 Craigpark
Denniston
Glasgow G31 2NA

Helen Sanderson
34 Broomfield Road
Heaton Moor
Stockport
Cheshire SK4 4ND

For 1 day workshops contact
Jane Harrison
at the address above

or Judy Ruddle
4 High Farm Close
Carlton
Stockton On Tees
Cleveland
TS21 1AN

or

Julie Lunt
The Firs
1 Barrswood Road
New Milton
Hampshire
BH25 5HS

The Aromatherapy Organisations Council
The A.O.C. is the governing body for the aromatherapy profession in the U.K. It is composed of both aromatherapy associations and training organisations, but does not have individual membership. The A.O.C. has its own constitution and is democratically governed. For further information and a list of recognised schools and colleges please send a S.A.E. to:

The Secretary
A.O.C.
3 Latymer Close
Braybrooke
Market Harborough
Leicestershire LE16 8LN

Index